# Strangers In My Mind

## Living with Post-Natal Psychosis

Rachel Day

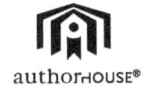

authorHOUSE®

*AuthorHouse™ UK Ltd.*
*500 Avebury Boulevard*
*Central Milton Keynes, MK9 2BE*
*www.authorhouse.co.uk*
*Phone: 08001974150*

*First published by AuthorHouse 4/13/2009*

*ISBN: 978-1-4389-7172-8 (sc)*

*This book is printed on acid-free paper.*

For the most wonderful gift God has ever given me, my daughter, Demi Day

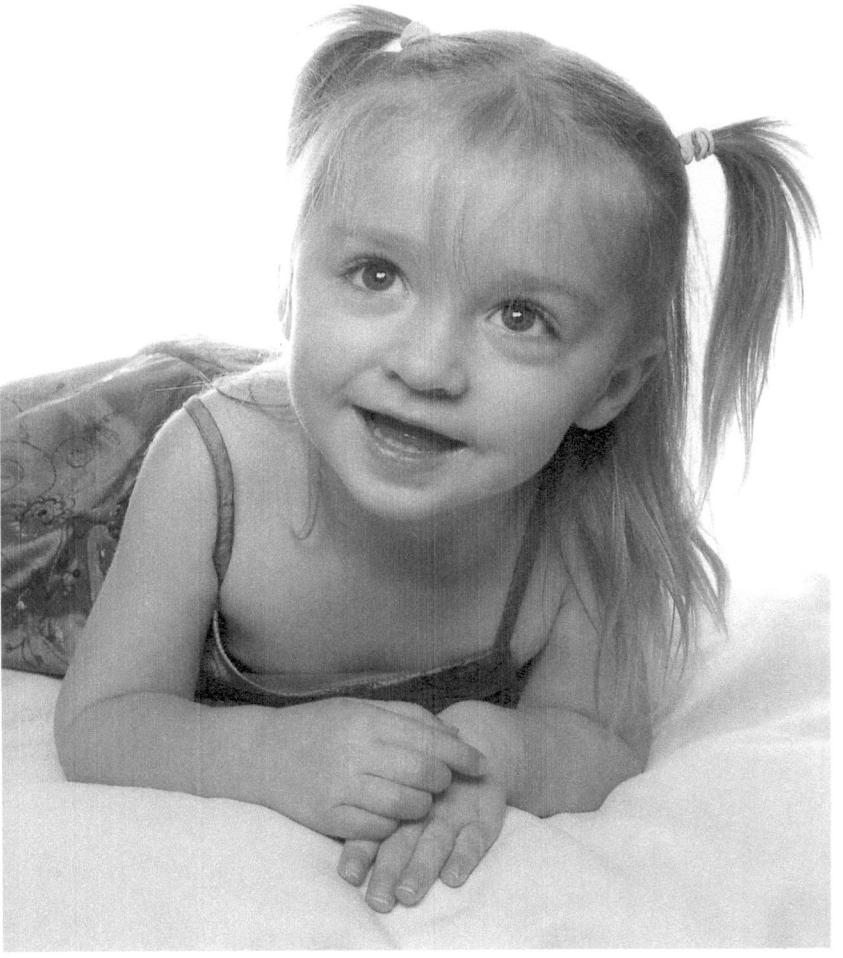

I would like to dedicate this book to my family.
To my parents, Celia and Philip.
To my sister, Joanna.
To my husband, and the love of my life; Dino Day.
And to my pride and joy, my son Scotty.

# August 2006

I can hear him banging on the door but I'm not bothered 'cause I know he can't get in. My phone's ringing, but it's on silent so I'm just ignoring it. I don't want to talk to him either. It doesn't matter if I close my eyes or keep them open, it's still pitch black with the light off and the blind drawn.

It's freezing on the cold tiles but I like feeling my body shiver and my lungs fill with the fresh air. That way I know I'm alive.
Demi's not making a sound, but I know she's staring at me. She's wide awake; listening to my heavy breathing and my sobs through the floodfuls of tears. Part of me wants to hold her; draw her into my arms and squeeze her; make her part of me. But I can't do that. I can't let her touch me; if I did that, I'd make her ill too.

He's found his keys, but the door won't budge. I did the right thing putting the drawers behind it. By the time he gets in the flat it'll be too late. I can hear him calling to me; he's talking to me, trying to get me to move the drawers, but I'm not coming out of the bathroom, I'm not turning back now.

I'm listening to everything; but I don't seem to be taking

1

it in. My phone's flashing again in the dark; Dad. I want to talk to him now, but I still can't answer it. I don't want to speak; if I whisper the whole building will hear me.

Dino's pushing the door, I can hear the drawers moving and now I'm starting to panic. I wasn't ready yet. I haven't had enough time. I'm shovelling the tablets in. I don't even have any water, my mouth is so dry and it feels like I'm choking while I'm trying to swallow.

My mind is spinning and I feel dizzy and sick; I'm heaving but I force my throat to close.
I've done it. Now I can breathe.
I don't feel cold now; my chest feels hot. I don't need to cry any more; soon it will all be over.
Now I'm not going to make her sick any more. I can hold her. My baby.
She's still quiet; though she can see me now. The glow from my flashing phone is lighting up her face. She's fixing her big knowing eyes on mine. I don't want to look at her; I can't bear her to see me like this any longer. I kiss her cheek and lay her back down. She still gazes up at me though; with her eyes that say more than words ever could.
She's the only one that knows. She can see into my soul; it talks to hers. She understands how I feel, that's why she's lying there now; letting me do this; 'cause she knows it's right.

I turn away from her stare and the tears return.
Now I'm gagging and choking; my body wants to vomit but I'm not going to let it.

I can still hear Dino; he's on the phone to my Dad now. They're downstairs; outside the flat. Oh no. I didn't want anyone to come yet; I didn't want anyone here 'til it was over.

My phones stopped flashing now and I'm panicking again. Dad. My Daddy; I need to talk to you.
He rings again and this time I answer. I'm trying to talk but I can't speak. My throat's sewn up; my voice box is suffocating with the evil that's inside me.
"Daddy..." It's all I can manage.
I don't want to tell him how I feel. I don't want anyone to know that I'm poisoned inside.
He knows I'm listening though and he tells me he loves me. "Don't be sad poppet...don't do anything silly. We love you; Dino loves you; Demi loves you." I can't listen any more. I have to hang up.

All of a sudden, my heart is aching. It hurts to feel these things. Why are all my senses now so strong; where had they gone?? I can smell the toilet; I didn't realise how close my face was to the dirty bowl. My stomach's retching and before I know it, I've puked up all the pills I'd taken hoping to end everything.

Dino's in the flat now; banging on the bathroom door, begging me to let him in and then it's open and I'm in his arms. Sobbing and shivering. He's kissing me and holding me tight, and I remember why I fell in love with this man.
He smells fresh from the outside air; Demi's kicking her legs with excitement and he talks to her; picks her up and

3

pulls her into our embrace, and suddenly it doesn't seem the same anymore.

This baby; my baby; the one that caused me all my pain and sorrow; suddenly she's a different baby. She's smiling at her Daddy and the light's on and the room's spinning and Dino won't let go of me; just draws my face into his chest and starts singing. Singing to Demi; singing to me. Humming to make my pain disappear.

And then I'm in bed. And it's dark again, but I'm not cold, I'm under the covers; wrapped up and warm. Dino's sitting on the bed, he's stroking my hair. I think he's put Demi to bed. Thank God, I can't bear to have her near me. If she see's me like this she might explode with the pain.

Dreaming; then I'm dreaming. I'm at the water front, and I can see the orange petals in the ocean; each one representing the hollow pain I feel inside, the babies that died inside me.

Dino and Demi are on the sand; they don't look sad like I do though. They look happy and Demi is playing with a sand castle.

Dino's laughing, and then he looks over at me and his smile fades. That's how it's been since the day I had her; his smile fading when he turns to me.

# March 2005

I think I'm having a mental breakdown; I'm confused, like I don't know who I am anymore.
I have to burn my brain, focus and remember who I am.
I know my name; Rachel Diana Day. I know I'm 23 and was born on April the second 1986. I know I've always lived in England, moving house every few years with my parents for Mum's work.

I know I have a little sister called Joanna who's now 20, who has two children, Ady and Franky with my husband's brother Skip.
I know all these things 'cause they are facts; things people have told me, recounted for me.

I faintly remember playing in the street with all the other children when I was about ten years old. I remember cuddling a tiny girl on my lap; her bones were frail and weak and she didn't grow like the rest.
I know I held her close to me; tight, but not tight enough to damage her. She was too fragile to squeeze.
I remember that day; because it's so significant to the person I think I am. I think that may have been the day my maternal desire began.
A new feeling of desperation inside me; craving what I

was far too young to have.

I know I had pets; lots of them. Tiny rodents I could protect and look after. I know I took home a half dead field mouse one day. Dad said the cat had got hold of it and that it would probably die.

I couldn't let that happen though; so I nursed it, for four days and four nights.

I remember feeding him droplets of milk from the tip of my tiny fingers and stroking his soft silky fur; holding him on my chest as I lay down, my heart bursting with adoration.

I made him a little bed and put leaves and hay in for him to sleep on.

Dad said he was too tiny to survive, because his eyes hadn't even opened and he was very small; just like a newborn baby; torn away from his mother; isolated and alone; probably terrified.

I called him Lucky.

It must have been the summer holidays though, because on the fifth day I had to go back to school.

Lucky needed to stay on his own for the whole eight hours I was away.

I put him a little bowl of milk in and made sure no-one could hurt him, but apparently it wasn't enough, because when Dad picked me up from school, he had the misfortune of breaking the bad news to me that Lucky had gone.

I felt so guilty; I had left him, abandoned him like I never should have.

He was a baby; he needed me to be there because he couldn't find his real Mummy.

I know it tore me up inside when he died, like I'd lost something far more precious than to everyone else he had seemed.

However, I think I was a pretty normal child.
I know I stole a £5 note from my Dad's wallet one day. He knew it had gone, and he probably knew it was me. He didn't confront me and humiliate me though. He said to Jo and I that whoever had taken it, had a few minutes to put it back, so when his back was turned I ran straight back with it, utterly ashamed of myself. I loved my Daddy for not hurting me, the way it must have hurt him for me to have taken it.

I got normal grades at school; didn't really excel in anything. Loved English and Music; played the flute and avoided Gym. I had a few close friends, but was never really considered the 'popular' type. I didn't mix with the crowd; I wanted to be me.
That's why I'm finding it so hard now. That all those years I stood up for my beliefs and didn't go popping pills with all my mates, or shagging boys behind the bushes like the other girls did. And now I don't really remember that girl.
I know Mum worked away all day; I don't really remember her in the few childhood memories I have. I know she took me shopping each weekend; showered me with clothes and toys; spoiling me, perhaps trying to justify the many hours we had missed together.

It always seemed to be Dad. Dad I'd run to when my chest hurt from my heart murmur, or when my head was banging with dizziness from the double vision I permanently suffer with; he who took me to hospital; numerous times in those teenage years.

He who caught me at the bottom of the stairs when had he not insisted on standing there for me, I may have broken my neck.

And I know I was running, running on the landing, running on the top few steps, tripping and flailing like a bird may fall when hurt, and I was just flying, soaring towards him, and then I was there, in his arms, both of us in shock, panting from the suddenness and that he held me really tight, like he never wanted to let go.

That wasn't the first time he'd saved my life as a child. I know I choked a few years later on a hardboiled sweet I'd insisted on having. I ran right past him to my Mum because I couldn't speak and I thought she would know what was happening. But he was up and he was running and he knew by the look in my eyes and then his arms were around me and they were squeezing me, pounding through my chest, forcing the air in my lungs and the sweet that clogged my throat to come tumbling out, and then I

sank to my knees, breathless, absolutely terrified, and I knew right then, from that very moment, but that he would never, ever, let anything hurt me.

I know for two years I lived a life of lies with a boyfriend I didn't love and grew only to despise. I remember feeling hatred seep from his eyes when he forced himself to look at me and knew from that moment on I could only be seen as ugly and worthless.

I know I finished school and studied Childcare at college. I worked hard on my Diploma and spent months working on assignments and in schools with little children I would quickly grow to love and then have to leave.

I remember being fourteen. Fourteen years old; a big girl by now, but a virgin when most of my friends were pro's at random, casual sex. And I'm kneeling beside this little boy with fair hair who I've spent the last two weeks with, six hours a day, drowning in the tears that are falling from his cheeks and I feel my insides hurting like my body can't accept I have to leave him. I remember that day because he was the first, but now I know there are so many more. I always have to leave my little boys eventually. The pain never eases, even after all these years.

My first job from college was in a special needs school for children with autism. My interview had been on my eighteenth birthday, I wore a gold chain around my neck with 18 on it and a polka dot skirt which my friends used to laugh at.

I remember my first day like it was yesterday. Sitting in the corner on a tiny blue chair; watching these children around me; every one of them disturbed. And then it dawns on me, and there's a lump in my throat and my eyes are watering; I'm crying where my heart is so full of sadness and pain and I just want to run; run away.

But I don't. Because I can't. I can't leave them, like I left the fragile little girl that used to curl up on my lap in the wind, or the little mouse I left to die alone.

So instead I stay, and I vow never to leave. Spending my days working with them; boys that don't see the world like I do.

I know too at 19, I sat in my Dads lounge with Dino. Terrified of what I was about to say.

"I think I love you." waiting, silently for his response.

My heart was beating faster as the seconds seemed to drag on for hours, but then he was holding my hand, kissing me; our first kiss. And I know I'm right. I knew I loved him the moment I met him. I told him how I felt before his lips had ever even touched mine, and I know he felt it back, confirmation etched in my heart as he pulled me in to him, telling me he loved me too, like he'd never loved another soul.

And soon, six weeks later, he was on his knees in our little bedroom, holding a box out to me, a beautiful diamond ring, and his hands are shaking and his lips are stumbling over words he is trying to say so perfectly and my arms are round his neck, pulling him on to the bed with me, smiles spread over our faces as I've never felt a moment like this before, a euphoric feeling swamping my body with sheer happiness that this man wants me to marry him, become his wife; for life.

*****

He's crying and he's screaming and he's forcing his shoes and his clothes off like the material is scraping at him, ripping his skin like fine blades, so I don't force them back on; I don't insist he wears them. Instead, I take them from him and place them on the floor beside me, and I think for a moment he doesn't understand, because normally they re-dress him, but I'm not going to, because I wonder if him seeing this, seeing me understand, will get through to him.

He looks up at me. His tiny body breathing now like it should be. And his eyes stare deep in to mine; though I know he isn't connecting with me, the same way I am with him.

So I sit down in front of him and cross my legs the way he has, and reach my hands out to his. I don't expect him to take them; sometimes human contact can be too much for him to bear. But I wait, and I watch to see if he is focusing.

I can see him rocking, moving his torso forwards and backwards, and then I touch him; rest my hand on top of his.
And he stops. Like something nasty crept out of his head, but he hasn't withdrawn his fingers like I thought he might. He's just watching me, waiting for my next move.

So I take the other one and hold them very gently in front of me.
"It's ok. You don't have to wear your clothes if they hurt you." I say softly, and he smiles at me, a cheeky smile where half his milk teeth are gone and he stares into my eyes for a moment, before he is off, up and running; tearing away from me.

*****

Why am I bleeding? People don't bleed when they're pregnant; do they? I'm shaking my head; but I know why I'm bleeding.

I shout down the stairs to my mum and she just stares at me. She knows; we both know. My heart is pounding and I keep shaking my head. I turn the shower on to the hottest temperature and practically crawl in.

It's burning me; scalding my skin, but I don't care.

Maybe it will make the pain go away; make all the nasty red between my thighs disappear so I can ignore what is happening; because deep down, I know.

She's calling back up to me, telling me to get out 'cause we need to go to the hospital. I can't move though, I can't stop scrubbing at my skin. I'm washing every inch of my body, denying that I'm losing my baby. My first baby. The baby we so desperately wanted.

They're pushing the probe inside me; they want to make sure; they need to know if my baby is ok. But it's not; it's dead. It died inside me. My body rejected it.

They try and tell me nicely, and I know the women are being kind and trying not to hurt me, but it's already done; my heart is already broken.

I felt it tear in two the minute I saw the screen. No heartbeat. My baby was gone.

They need to take blood now; to check I'm ok. But I don't care. I don't care if I'm ok; I just want my baby back.

I turn my face away from the needle; my arm might as well be severed from my body because right now I can't feel a thing.

I'm focusing on a picture; it's beautiful. The light on the sand is drifting me away; saving me from this hollow feeling inside.

That's when I decide that's where it is.
The baby isn't dead and flushed down the toilet to the sewers; it's in the ocean; swimming with all the tropical fish; basking in the sunshine; calm and alive.

*****

Dino is holding me in his arms; so tight it hurts but I don't care. We're both sobbing; uncontrollably. No-one else can see us now though; we're in bed at home. It's so quiet, like we're missing a sound we never heard.

My tummy's in agony and I've got my arms wrapped round it; trying to protect what's already gone.
We can't even speak, but then, there's nothing either of us can say to make anything better.
It's really just the beginning of the pain we are about to experience.

*****

*Who wants to talk about a baby that's not here,*
*Who wants to listen to me re-live all my fears?*
*Who remembers her like I do,*
*Who can see her face, her pretty eyes she never looked through?*
*He can't ignore the truth, pretend it never happened,*
*He seems to think, that will stop him being saddened.*
*Just babies ourselves, too young for it to work,*
*Our child who was once alive, stolen, from us, he took her.*
*She didn't even live a minute, nor take her first breath,*
*All because it was our fate, for her, we will always miss.*
*I see the other babies and I wish she was still here,*

*So when she cried or whimpered I could hold her near.*
*But this is all impossible; it's all completely unforgettable,*
*And she's gone from my arms forever.*
*I miss her dark brown hair and her glossy stare,*
*Her still dark eyes, fixed forever, onto mine,*
*Wishing I could hold her just one last time.*
*I sit by her grave, crying empty tears,*
*Wondering how my life will change, over all the coming*
*years.*
*I stare at her name, engraved on the stone,*
*Wishing I could pick her up and take her home.*
*But that will never be,*
*As she's not meant to be with us,*
*God planned out my life and she's gone because he needs*
*her, up in Heaven.*
*I just hope she can see me, when I lie down at night,*
*Thinking of my baby that's now no-where in sight.*
Confused; I'm so confused. What life did I live before
this sadness?

# May 2005

I can't get out of bed. I can't physically get the strength to drag myself up. I can't remember the last time I washed; or ate; or slept. I can't think about anything, except them.

Dino comes and goes, work and sleep, work and sleep... I know he tries to talk to me, but I can't focus on anything he says. I need to stay in bed; I need to curl up and hide away.

I think about my babies every day; sometimes all day.
I didn't want to go through it again; I didn't want to feel that pain, the hollow feeling that never goes away.
But I did.
For some reason; I had to lose 3 more.

I'd been so happy. I'd fallen pregnant again so quickly. I was jumping up and down when I saw the test read positive. I couldn't stop smiling and I thought it would be different this time.
But not for me. It wasn't meant to be; or so people kept telling me.

I felt the twinges in my back again, and saw the pink stain on my knickers while I was at work. I had to leave; I had to get out of there. I had to run and be home. Hide away

and pretend this was NOT happening to me again!
I couldn't hide for long though, because before long, the babies were coming out. Three, dead tiny babies.

\*\*\*\*\*

I'm back at the hospital; and I have to walk back to the car to go home.
I know he's waiting there for me; watching me coming. Searching my face for an answer.
The truth is, my heart is breaking inside, like it's bleeding and seeping pain through my entire body.
I'm trying not to cry though.
I'm trying to be strong, at least until I'm at home hiding, alone.

But when I get in to the car, I only have to look at him and he knows.
"Oh Daddy..." And then my eyes are burning and stinging and I can hardly control my breathing.
He just grabs my hand; grips it so tight, like that pain will erase any other.
And his eyes are shining in the sunlight; glowing and glossy, speaking so much to me; no words are necessary.

There's a silent pause while he brings me in close to him; holding me against his chest so he can contain my grief.
"I'm sorry pet. It's ok. Your time will come..." and he trails off because there's nothing else he can say, and nothing else I want to hear.
And I know his eyes are leaking; he isn't crying, he doesn't cry, his eyes are just watering with sadness for me.
Because Daddy knows my grief; he's lived it with me.

*****

Dino says it's an obsession.

It's my fifth pregnancy test this month and I'm standing still; breathless; silently praying.

He keeps telling me not to get my hopes up and right now I just want to shut him out.

My entire life is now focused on getting pregnant again.

I lock the bathroom door behind me and relish in the excitement of what could be.

I know time's up and I can look now. But part of me is too afraid. I don't want to turn to it yet; in case it's blank again.

In the seconds that follow, my mind has opened and I imagine rushing from the room and throwing my arms around Dino.

I'm tapping my feet on the cold tiles and swaying backwards and forwards.

I can't wait any longer and I spin round and snatch the stick up from the sink.

It's negative.

My stomach hurts, like I've just been punched.

I'm embarrassed now; so humiliated. 'Cause I've wasted more money, more time, more heart ache, and all for nothing.

I'm not going to cry; I'm not sad right now; just angry.

I clench my fists and leave the bathroom.

Dino looks over at me; waiting for a response, a reaction he can read.

I'm not even going to say it. I'm not even going to look at him. Not give him the satisfaction of being right; again.

He can tell though and he's not spiteful like I am. He walks over to me and puts his arms around me, and holds me tight, because he knows exactly how I'm feeling inside. But I just shrug away from the embrace and tell him that tomorrow the test will be different.

*****

They're both sitting there; rigidly and I'm worried of what is coming; scared something is really wrong; nerves tearing through me.

I'm waiting and waiting and the minutes seem to drag on for hours and then Mum just comes out with it and it's like a bolt of lightening sending thousands of shock waves through my body.

"Jo's pregnant." She blurts out and I turn from the end of the hallway where I'd paced just moments ago and I look back at her; stare right in to her eyes.

"If you're joking, if this is a joke….I swear to God…" And my lips have tightened and I can feel my heart thudding inside me, but she's shaking her head and holding her hands together, her body so stiff and her eyes are slightly damp, and my gaze turns to Jo; I can't move from this spot I can't even breathe, and I look in to her eyes and know it's true.

And in the seconds that follow, so many thoughts go through my mind and I realise that they're scared, they're worried of how I'll react and Jo's face looks covered with guilt, like they're sorry she is pregnant and not me. Like this will break me in two, and I can't do it.

So now I'm running, running up the hallway that seems never to end and I'm flinging my arms around her as she flinch's and she thinks I'm going to hit her, but of course

18

I'm not; I'm just holding her, squeezing her, kissing her and I feel so happy for her, like this is a wonderful time to celebrate and I can't let how my heart bleeds inside for my own baby ruin my little sisters first.

*****

*Mummy please don't cry now, there's no need to be sad,*
*I'm always with you, trust me, I'm who you'll always have.*
*I see you every day you know, I hear your silent tears,*
*I feel the pain you never show, I understand your fears.*
*Please don't be mad at Daddy, he's just a little scared,*
*Know he will always love us, and mention us in his prayers.*
*When you are sleeping in the night, I hear him call your name,*
*Wishing you could be beside him, to silently share the pain.*

# June 2005

I'm standing on the beach; staring out at the ocean. Watching the waves slide in and out; calming me; slowing my breathing.

Dino and I are holding the flowers; the orange roses he bought me to make me smile again.

I walk up to the edge of the water; feel it trickle over my toes, icy cold.

I don't want to throw them; I don't want it to be like I'm chucking them away.

So I walk in further and place them in the waves.


I'm not crying today. My eyes aren't red and sore now. They're dry; wide.

I'm thinking of the day I lost them. The day I lost my first little baby.

I couldn't accept it, I couldn't 'get over it' until we'd accepted them.

That's why we named them.

My first little baby; Leah.

She was so tiny; just born before her time.

Wrapped in her thick little sac; protecting her like my body couldn't.

And my triplets. The babies my body 'rejected'; Ashley, Aaliyah, Adrienne.

And suddenly they're real; more real this moment than I

felt when I bore them.

Dino is holding me; drawing me in to him.
He's crying now too; because this moment is real for him.
He doesn't feel the dull ache inside him like I do; like there's a deep hole that should be filled right now; where my babies should be growing.

I'm stroking the soft petals of the last rose. I'm too afraid to let it go.
Dino holds my hand and I muster the inner strength to push it away.
I have to watch them all floating; I can't leave just yet.
The beach is deserted; the sand and the water and this secret moment left just for us.

And soon they are gone.
Swimming away from me; all together again; floating into the distance, all bound together by the same water; just swaying, and waiting for me to join them.

*****

Its 4am and I've woken up soaked in my own sweat. Dino's fast asleep next to me. I try and wake him but he's passed out from the alcohol he's drunk the night before.
I can see the stars and the moon shining through the window.
I am absolutely terrified. Something bad is going to happen; someone is going to kill me.

My heart is racing now, and I can't move for fear of

dying.

There's a man in the flat, with a knife, I just know it. He wants to kill me.

No, I'm wrong, there's a tsunami. It's coming to England, I'm in Bournemouth and the sea is right beside me. I close my eyes and see the giant waves coming over the buildings. I'm going to drown to death; my darling Dino is going to drown to death.

I have to ring my Dad; I need him to come and get us. We all need to be together if we are going to drown and die.

I can see myself dying; holding their hands, swallowing endless mouthfuls of water.

Dad answers the phone and listens to me gabble.

My breath has quickened and I'm panicking. I need to get up and move Dino. We need to get out before the water smashes the windows right above us.

Dad calms me down. He says there isn't going to be a tsunami in England. There is nobody in the flat besides me and Dino. I wish he could wake up and tell me that himself.

I'm sure I can hear breathing outside the door; I just know there's someone after me.

Dad's right though; no tsunami, not tonight anyway.

I'm too tired by the end of the phone call and eventually drift back off to sleep, only to be woken by the reminder of the ocean; the water diving towards us, covered in orange rose petals, just like the ones we threw into the sea in memory of the babies we lost.

It's beautiful though; just so painfully sad.

*****

Back at the water; the sun beating down on me, my arms are bare and soaking in the sun. The sea is glistening, shimmering in the light and there's a boy flying a kite on the shore.

I'm watching him as if I know him; as if I recognise him from my father's memories; a boy; his son. Lying on the sand, letting the wind pull him along, flying the deep blue, diamond shaped kite so it just skims the sand before rising it back up again and turning with a smile.

And I'm mesmerised by him; like I'm seeing in to a chapter of their pasts, before I realise it isn't him at all, and that those moments are long gone.

# October 2005

It's gorgeous today; the sun is bright and warm and there isn't even a breeze.
I feel like I'm living a previous dream; but this time it's different.
I'm walking back to the car; I'm trying not to run.
I have to walk slowly; I have to take every step at minimum pace; carrying the precious cargo within me.
I reach the car and climb in.
Dad's staring at me; searching my eyes for emotions.
I know he can see the tears that have stained my cheeks; along with the black mascara, that's now strewn across my face.

"No heartbeat?" He asks me, squeezing my fingers, trying to keep me from crashing back down.
"No Daddy, there is..." and suddenly I can't speak; I'm just nodding and sobbing and I can hear him breathing out heavily; like he had to hold his breath for fear of jinxing it.
And then his cheeks are wet too and he can't stop smiling and he starts the engine so we can go home and tell Mum and Dino and I think my hands are shaking and I'm watching the clouds; talking to whoever's up there; thanking them; begging them to protect it.

*****

Suddenly I'm in a world I could only have dreamt of a year ago.
I'm a different girl now; a girl who's dreams have come true.
Dino's looking at the scan picture with me. We can hardly see the baby; it just looks like a tiny bean.
A kidney bean; that's the size it is right now; minute.

I'm reading the books again; the ones I put away after I lost the babies before.
I'm thinking about it growing inside me; my husbands' tiny baby; resting within me.
And then I feel it; a new love. Gushing through me; drowning my body in a new emotion I've not felt before.
Because this time it's real; this time I'm not going to distance myself.
I'm going to love it; because that way, if love alone can protect it, it will never be harmed.

*****

The water is clear again; blue-green, twinkling in the light of the sun and Dad and I are back; sitting at the Head this time; watching the men with their little fishing boats, rowing out ever so slowly, beckoning the fish to them, and Dad turns to me and says "Tight Lines.." and smiles, 'cause he says that's what fishermen always say to one another.
And then he's flashed back, to the world he lived before, and he's telling me of a boat he made and painted, with

his first born sons name along the side and how he used to float it in the water; carefully watching it, so as not to lose it, like eventually his son would come to lose him.

# November 2005

It's my wedding day; our wedding.
My dress is beautiful, no frills, no train. Just simple; because that's all it needs to be for us.

I know my sister dreams of a beautiful wedding. I don't desire that at all though.
I desire the baby I now feel growing inside of me.

It's freezing outside, the wind blowing my curled hair about my face.
My Father is here, my Daddy, the man I could never compare another love to.
And he's walking me in; through the double doors for everyone to see.
And I've never felt so proud. He's not got his stick today; he's walking alone, except for his arm linked through mine, like it will always be.

And then I see him.
My darling Dino. The man I am about to make my husband.
Suddenly it's like no-one else is in the room. It's just us.
I go to him and we say our vows which are traditional in this beautifully small decorated registry office room.

Then the ring is on my finger, soon to be placed with the diamond ring he bought me six months before and his hand is on mine and I see his eyes are bright and colourful today, wet with tears of joy; same as mine and my Fathers.

He looks so handsome in his suit. Absolutely gorgeous; charming, a man I've not seen in this light before. And I'm so happy. Like nothing could spoil how I'm feeling inside.

I carry his baby behind the satin ivory gown and his heart on my finger in the form of a gold band and I smile, a genuine smile, that cannot fade now, because I know that for the rest of my life, he will be with me, our hearts joined forever, our souls,

unbreakable and when he says 'For better or for worse... in sickness and in health...' I know he means it; really, truly means it; just like I do.

And then it's evening, and we're dancing in the dark. The reception room is empty in my head; just us dancing, a song that says it all for us... Power of Love.

'Because I am your lady....and you are my man....whenever you reach for me.....I'll do all that I can...'

I can feel myself melt in his arms and I never want this moment to end.

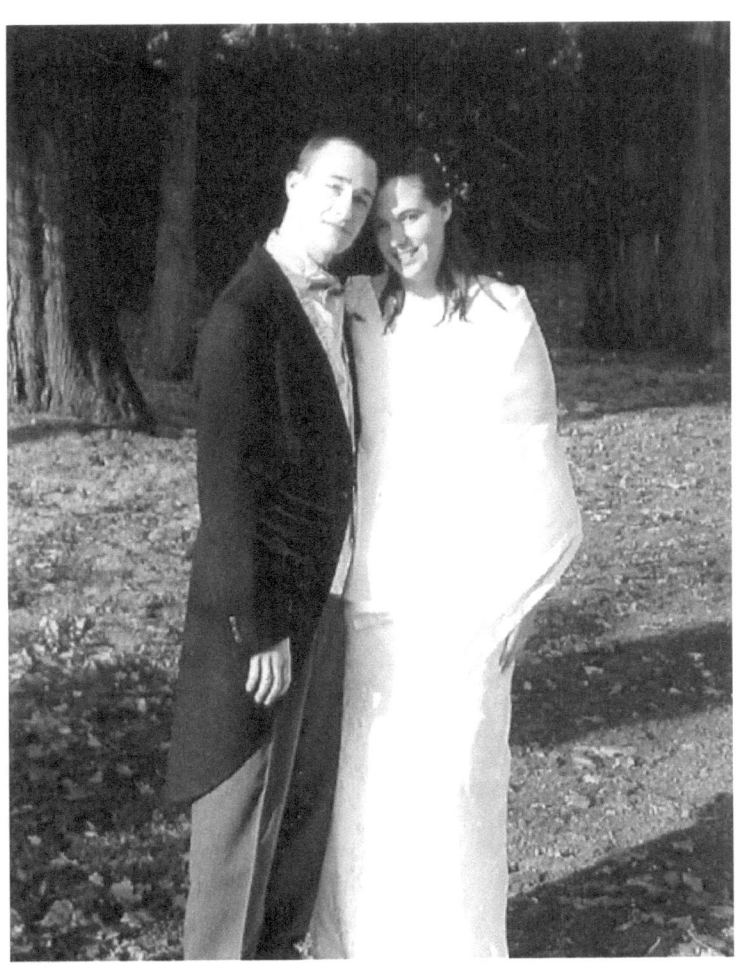

My darling Dino and I

# January 2006

Oh Thank God. There's still a heartbeat! I'm five months pregnant and there is still a heartbeat.

"It's a girl" the pretty Indian woman smiles at us as we leave the ward.
I can't wipe the smile from my face; I think it's stuck there. I've never felt so wonderful. Never before, have I experienced the feeling that's over powering my body.

Dino's got his arm around me and he squeezes me into him. I'm so happy I could burst and the smile on his face just melts me.
I need to tell everyone I know; I need to tell the whole world that I am carrying my husband's baby girl and that she is alive.

We're going to call her Demi. Dino chose it; he loves it. It's perfect.
I don't want her to have a middle name though, because Dino doesn't have one. I need our daughter to be just like him; I want her to love him the way I've always loved my Daddy.

*****

I'm folding up the hundreds of tiny bodysuits we've bought the baby. Some are a pale pink, some lilac or yellow or green. I wanted to get a big variety of colours for her; bright colours so her heart can shine as bright as her clothes will. They are all lined up, pressed perfectly in the drawers we've kept just for her.

The top, covered in beautiful ornaments, crystal baby shoes with pink bows and a tiny hairbrush and comb set I want to use so delicately on her fine strands. Her box is beside them, a purple box with a ribbon tying the covers together; all the scan pictures enclosed, alongside special letters I've written her. Everything is just lying perfectly, waiting, as I am, for her arrival.

# May 2006

My waters have broken and I'm so excited.

We're exhausted; tired from the late night before. The stress of it still pressing down on me.

Dino sits bolt upright now though.

He just stares at me; his eyes wide with wonder and excitement.

I can't stop smiling; and suddenly I'm up; rushing about; grabbing everything I think I need, because I'm not ready; it's too early.

We need to go to Southampton. We need to be there so they can help the baby when she's born. Look after whatever it is they found with her last week.

I'm not even thinking about that though; I'm just thinking how excited I am; and how I can't wait to hold her.

It's been four days. Four long, tiring days of waiting.

She isn't ready; she shouldn't be here yet.

She must have been scared the night my waters broke; the noise and the confusion must have worried her.

Hearing me crying and screaming; feeling my chest rise and fall with fear.

So now we're waiting. Dino and I, at the hospital she is to be born at.

He can stay with me most nights; but we're both so tired.

The nurses keep asking me for blood and are monitoring

us. I just want to sleep.

Induced, what does induced mean? Why does it hurt so much more than my sisters labour seemed to? I need to have the epidural; I need the pain to go away.

What's a catheter?

I can't handle this pain. I need the gas and air so I can fade away from it all; and then it's there, and I'm floating, and I've lost all my senses, like I can't feel anything or hear anything; and all that exists is me and the tube in my mouth.

Like sucking the gas in, is all that matters in my entire life. Like if I stop I'll die and I'll be forced away from this amazing new feeling.

I've never done any drugs before, and the feeling of this alien toxin inside me; just melts me completely.

I don't have any limbs anymore; or a body from the neck down. Just a mouth; that's all that I am.

I don't have a head or eyes or ears. There's just blackness and silence.

I can feel something like a chest rising and falling, but I know there isn't one there.

Suddenly someone's taken it away, and now my alien world disappears and pain is slicing through me, the body I wished I didn't have again.

People are looking at me; Jo is there, Dino I think and women I don't know.

"Noooo!!" I'm screaming, I'm begging them to give it back, but they won't.

I can't talk; I can't even look straight. I need to keep my eyes closed; I need to hold on to the blackness because it's all I have left from the pain free world I wish I could retreat to.

Why are there so many people around me?
I've been pushing for hours; I don't even know how. I can't feel anything from the epidural.
I just want the gas and air back, but the women won't let me.
I'm so exhausted, I haven't slept for 36 hours and all I want to do is close my eyes and not wake up.

Jo thrusts a piece of paper in front of me.
I'm begging her to get me a c-section.
I don't want to sign it, whatever it is, I don't want to, take it away.
But she won't, and now I'm forced to look at her and her eyes seem to be screaming at me, so I just grab the pen and scribble something down, and then it's gone and there's a woman in front of me.
She's telling me I need some help and that they're going to use forceps and cut me.
Cut me?? Oh Jesus no...I can see Jo's eyes shut tightly and now I'm terrified.
But the woman is doing it and she says the baby is there and I need to push when she tells me so that all the pain can stop, and then I can, like my body isn't hurting anymore, I've just floated away from the pain, and then she's here, lying on my chest, staring up at me crying and I can't take my eyes off Dino, I can't stop looking at him, because I love him so much and I can never thank him enough for giving me this precious gift.

She doesn't need an operation, does she? Can she breathe ok? Why is there a huge lump on her neck?

I can't see straight. My body is so full of drugs; there are wires stretching from me to drips and needles; I think I'm going to be sick.

Jo's there, holding my hand like I held hers when her baby was born. She was 17 and braver than I am now.

I can't help vomiting. It's bright green. My sick is bright green and I grimace at the sight of it. Jo says it's ok, and it's just the drugs that have made me feel so ill.

I want to see my baby; can she breathe?


I can hear her crying; she's screaming and crying and all I want to do is hold her.

And then she's in my arms, and Dino's holding us both and I can see her eyes, her little face peering over the blanket that's wrapped around her. She's ok. She can breathe. She's just got this awful liquid filled lump on her neck.

They tell me it's a cyst, so I cover it up and hide what's disfiguring my perfect bundle.

She stops crying and she just looks up at me, and my eyes are streaming and I can't see through the tears and the dizziness.

Dino has to take her as I think I'm so weak I could drop her.

I know they're stitching me up but I think I'm going in and out of consciousness.

I can hear people fussing around me, and see Jo wince as she's watching what their doing between my legs.

Dino can't look.

I can hear my parents outside. Mum comes in and smiles at me. I think she's talking but I can't hear her.

My head hurts and I feel sick again. I don't want anyone to touch me. I just want my baby girl to breathe.

*****

Why are other women getting up and walking around? Demi's lying next to me; crying for some milk. I can't get the strength to pick her up though. My arms are like jelly.

The epidural wore off days ago, but I still can't move. My legs permanently have pins and needles and it feels like I'm drained of all the energy I once had.

Is this how it's supposed to feel when you've just had a baby? I can't sit, because my stitches are in agony. I can't even move to go to the toilet. I'm terrified I fall over or my wee stings too much.

A woman who had a c-section is just leaving; she looks so happy and full of life. What's going on?

I feel so alone; I need someone to come and see me; to hug me.

People are sitting up, doing puzzles, laughing, talking. I don't have the energy to do any of those things.

I try and pick Demi up during the night for a feed and nearly drop her. I've buzzed for help but I think the nurses want me to do it myself. Why can't they see I physically can't??

I'm using all my energy just to live right now. I try and

lie in the same position all day, because if I turn or move then I get some sort of head rush and my mind starts spinning.

The nurses keep opening the curtains but I want them closed; I don't want anyone to look at us. I don't want any of the other women to see how weak and incapable I am; or see Demi's cyst when all their babies are perfect.

Just hide us; please.

\*\*\*\*\*

They said I need a blood transfusion. I'm so scared. Does that mean my body hasn't got enough blood now? What if I bleed to death?

I hate the needles, I'm full of them. A drip for something, I don't even know what, a different one for the blood. I hate seeing this big bag of blood hanging beside me. I want to rip it from my arm. I don't want anyone else's blood inside me. I feel sick again.

I need a wee.

I've got to drag myself to the toilet and bring the stupid drip along with me. I can hear the trolley thing wheeling beside me.

My wrist is hurting every time I move it and I'm scared I pull the wire out.

God, I think I'm going to collapse. I just make it to the toilet and then I think I pass out while sitting on it.

No-one knows I'm in here.

Where is everyone? Where are Jo and Dino? I need them to come back but I know it's so far.

I'm awake again; I need to go back to bed. Is it cold? I feel so very cold. I think my jaw is juddering.

I've got to get back to my bed.

I think I've got 3 blankets over me; I'm so cold, or am I?
Why are my teeth chattering?
The lady opposite me must be able to hear them. She
keeps asking if I'm ok. Of course I'm ok, aren't I? You're ok,
you've had a baby, and surely I'm ok; I think, nodding.
Now my whole body is shaking. I'm not imagining it am
I? My teeth won't stop chattering. I try and stop my face
from moving. I can't. It's annoying me. It's my mouth
and I want it to stop; but it won't.
She asks me again if I'm ok. I smile and nod at her; I like
her; she's had a baby boy; she looks happy.

I'm so cold. I press the buzzer; I want to ask for another
blanket.
Someone comes and I try and ask for another cover but
my jaw is chattering so much I can't speak.
Before I know what's happening she's disappeared.
Now there are four women around me, or five. I can't count
them; I can't even see them all. What's happening?
Someone's just yanked the wire from my arm. I want to
scream at them not to do that! I don't want to bleed to
death; don't do that! But I can't speak; my whole body is
convulsing now.
I keep glancing at my baby girl. She can't see me can she?
She can't see what's happening to me? Not at three days
old, please?!

Then there's a weird mask over my face; and a tank of
something next to me; it looks like the gas and air I had
days ago and I think oh good something to stop me

feeling like this, but it's not and it doesn't feel the same and suddenly I realise I've got an oxygen mask over my face.

OXYGEN!? Why have I got an oxygen mask on??

They're putting needles in me again; they want my blood. I've lost enough. Leave my blood alone.

There's a new drip in my other arm; what the hell's going on?

It's water. Someone says they're flushing the blood out. It wasn't right for me.

What the hell are they saying? I can't hear them anymore.

I'm just breathing; breathing in the oxygen. I don't know why, I can breathe by myself.

Suddenly it's my wedding day again and I can see Dino and I dancing. He's got his arms around me and I'm stroking the back of his head. We're both smiling and spinning. Everyone is there but I can't focus on them; just on my husbands face.

And then I see the water; the ocean I always love to see. I can see the orange rose petals floating on the surface, where we threw them years ago. And I can hear babies laughing.

Then I'm spinning again in the dark at my wedding reception and everything goes black.

Now it's gone and I'm back in this horrible room. I can see women drawing my curtains and someone's gone to see the woman with the baby boy. She looks scared but I'm trying to smile at her.

I can see Demi next to me; she's quiet now but I think she's awake; watching, listening.

Suddenly I'm moving. My bed is being wheeled away. Oh God, No! My baby, I try and scream; don't take me away from my baby.
It's ok though; she's coming with me. They're bringing my baby; thank God.
And then a woman asks me who I want her to call? Why do I need her to call someone? Dino I say; or my Dad. I just want my family. Tell them to come here, please?!

Now I'm in another room; it's totally different. I wake up and wonder where the hell I am?
There are no other women with babies; just me and my baby girl and a lady who's sitting next to us.
I'm completely naked; I've got drips from both arms. I think I need a wee, but when I try and stand up I just wet the bed and the floor. Why did that happen? I did NOT tell my body to wee yet! I'm so embarrassed. I just want to crawl back into bed and hide.
I can hardly move though.
I drag myself back into bed with the help of the woman that does not look too impressed at having to clean up my wee, and lie down flat on my back.
I close my eyes and try to sleep.

Suddenly I can hear my Dad coming down the corridor outside. He bursts into the room with my Mum by his side and starts shouting and swearing at all the women who are looking after me.
"If she fucking dies....if anything happens to her...I swear

to God...." He's got his angry face on. I guess to the women he looks pretty scary, but I know he won't hurt a fly.

I grimace at my Mum and she tries to take him out the room. I can still hear him shouting and I know he's close to tears. I'm trying to block out what he's saying, I'm not really going to die am I?

Is this what it feels like to be dying?

And then I see him. He's hiding in the dark I'm sure. My darling Dino. It's like he doesn't want to come near me incase breathing beside me will kill me.

I smile at him though my head is spinning and really I just want to die now.

His eyes are welling up and he holds my hand. It feels like he's crushing the life from me though, like any blood left inside me will squirt out of an open needle wound.

I have to pull away and I just close my eyes and try to disappear.

*****

I look at her lying beside me. Her eyes are closed and she looks so tiny and frail. I wish I could talk to her like I can hear the other mothers doing to their babies.

I've drawn the curtains so nobody can see in. I've put my puzzle book down; it feels like the pen weighs a ton.

I watch her tiny chest moving with her breathing, her little fists clenched up to her sides.

I look at her and realise.............

I feel nothing.

*****

We're driving along, slowly round the bends, my newborn daughter strapped in carefully to the back of the car.

It's windy today, the breeze is flowing in through my open window and I'm watching the old women sitting on the bench, wondering what they are thinking and puzzling the lives they must have led.

And I find myself looking at them longer than we've past, till I'm staring at them through the rear-view mirror; questioning if any of them resemble my Great Gran-Gran, wondering, but never knowing, if they look anything like she did.

Soon though, they are tiny dots in the distance, and then we've turned the corner, on the road down to her house, and I'm staring at the window; the very top window, waiting and just hoping that I'll see her waving down towards us.

But his gaze has turned now and he's looking at another; a beautiful house beside it that looks so much prettier than hers, and he tells me that he remembers when it first got built and I think about the time then and how small he must have been.

# June 2006

## *Diagnosis*

Feeling very miserable, low or tearful for no apparent
reason
Irritability
Sleep disturbances
Affected appetite - weight gain/loss
Anxiety
Feeling worthless
Believe yourself to be failing as a parent
Increased fear/worries
Self loathing
Suicidal thoughts
Nightmares / horrible thoughts that can be disturbing
Thoughts of self-harming/harming your baby
Lack of interest in the baby or the care/hygiene of baby
or self
Losing interest in sex

I've just been asked to tick boxes which apply. They might
as well ask me to strip off and run around the surgery
screaming and skipping. How humiliating.
The doctor has the decency to turn away; but I can feel
my cheeks burning anyway.

My heart is racing and I can feel my head spinning when I close my eyes. It feels sore in my chest. I don't want to read these things; I don't want to see them printed in black and white; factual.

I can hear him writing something down; it feels like the sound of the pencil scribbling is going to burst my ear drums! Why are my senses so strong lately?
I want to scream at him to be quiet! I can't think straight while his pencil is making that awful noise.

I can't do it; my throat has gone dry and my hands are sweating.
I scrape the pen through each box, as quietly and as slowly as I can. The words are jumping out at me.... weight gain.....tearful.....nightmares....suicidal....
I put the paper down and turn myself away.
I squeeze my eyes shut and clench my fists under my thighs.

He takes the paper and adds some numbers up. He's scoring it I think.
I can't see him through my closed eye lids but I know his kind eyes are watching me.
He starts talking to me about PND - talks about it as if it's normal. I'm not alone...is he joking? Of course I'm alone. I feel like I've been stuck on another planet somewhere and I'm supposed to communicate with a new species... although what's funny is that I quickly realise that I am the new species.

He says I need to go on some tablets and that I will start

to feel better soon.

I try and look at him; but I can't keep eye contact for more than a few seconds. I am so embarrassed. I'm on pills because of my mental health state. I want to curl up and hide again and just fade away like a cloud.

The baby is next to me in her car seat. He starts questioning my relationship with her and I can feel myself start to panic. I don't want him to take my baby girl away; I don't want them to tell everyone I've failed as a mother and make me lose her.

I'm smiling now and gabbling on like an excited child.

He isn't smiling though. I'm pretty sure he can see right through me.

He wants to see me again in a few weeks if I'm not feeling any better.

I like this man; the same man that helped me when I lost my first baby. I quickly make a decision though; a promise to myself; I will never ever return to this surgery; I will never tell them of my 'condition'.

It needs to be a secret.

*****

Dino's back at work now and suddenly it feels like my whole world has come crashing down. I feel locked in this room. A tiny cell for me and my baby while my husband's out all day working. God, I resent him for that.

We're supposed to be staying here for a while but I can't bear the thought of being here. I hate it.

I need to go home. I need to go back to my Dads.

I crawl out of bed and swallow the happy pills the doctor has given me. So far, I don't feel very happy.

Demi's quiet; as always. She isn't crying; that only comes at night or when her tummy's hurting from the colic that grips at her.

I need to change her nappy, but I'm terrified. Nobody else understands how difficult this is. I see Jo change Ady's nappies every day and she doesn't make any fuss. I can't let anyone see me when I do her nappy. I can't let anybody see how distraught I get when I have to change her.

She's wearing the same clothes she wore yesterday and I think I need to change them as the neck line is all covered in dry milk.

I try and focus on something else while I'm doing it. It's using too much energy though and as soon as she's dressed I have to lie down for twenty minutes.

I forgot to take my iron tablet though and have to rummage through all the crap lying around to find where I threw them in rage the previous day.

I try not to gag as I swallow it; drinking from the manky water bottle I've got lying beside the bed.

I need to get up; I have to get out.

I take Demi downstairs; and suddenly I feel even worse. I'm in this house; this mans empty house. Dino's Dad is so kind to let us stay here and yet he doesn't understand that I see it only as my hell.

Demi's buggie is standing there where Dino left it yesterday. He always sorts her buggie out. He puts it in and out of the car; he moves it, he pushes it, he cleans it. I don't even want to look at it.

I put Demi in it and try to remember everything she is going to need for the whole day. I have no intention of coming back until Dino is home tonight.
I grab all the bottles that he made last night from the fridge and shove them in a carrier bag on the buggie handle. I grab my book and her nappies.
There is nothing else I need. Nothing else I could possibly want to take from this place.

I notice that our fridge stinks and desperately needs cleaning. I heave at the thought of it; though the smell could be worse.
"We're ready." I say, and she stares up at me with those big wise eyes of hers.
For half a second I smile, 'cause I know where we're going.
"Granddad!" I beam and I swear I see her lips twinge.

And then we're walking, and it's a gorgeous day. No matter how crap I feel inside; I cannot deny the beauty of the weather.
The sun is shining and there isn't a cloud in the sky, and for just a while, for the short walk there, I feel good.
Demi looks up at me the whole way. I think of all the different things I could say to her, but then people begin to walk past me and I don't want to speak to a baby that can't even understand what I'm saying.

And then I see it. I'd forgotten to cover it; her cyst.
I have to stop the buggy, I need to pull the side covers up,

47

and I don't want anyone to see it.

I grab a cardie of hers from underneath the buggy and wrap it round her. I have to do it up right to the collar and then put the blanket over her until it covers that side of her face.

It makes me want to shiver seeing it like that. I don't want people looking at it and pointing at her.

Sometimes it makes me feel like it's the most private part of her body. I don't care if people see her bits when they help do her nappy, but if they see her cyst, if their gaze changes even slightly then I feel like I want to scream.

And I watch them too; I watch their stares, just waiting to see it; so that inside I can remind myself why no one is ever coming near my baby, why nobody can ever see her like that and why I hate every single person that comes near her.

And then we're here. I'm finally here. A five minute walk feels like it's killing me inside. And my Daddy's here, waiting for our arrival, and I think I throw my arms around him, but only briefly because I'm too exhausted to cuddle.

Soon we're upstairs and Demi's in her crib beside my Dads side of the bed.

I have to lie on my Mums side; it makes me feel slightly closer to her. Though truth is, I've never felt so far away.

Demi's quiet. She's always quiet. I suddenly realise that she never makes any sounds.

I walk over to her cot and she looks so happy to see me.

She can't smile yet; but I know she wants to. I never peer over her cot; I never look in; I never speak to her.

"Hi." I manage, and she stares up at me. I have to shift my eyes and I concentrate on the hem of my t shirt for a minute.

I want to tell her I love her, but I utter "Go to sleep" and rise from that side of the bed.

Still she is quiet, and this concerns me now. It dawns on me that I never speak any more. Certainly not to her. She probably doesn't understand that as people we speak.

I try and push this thought out of my head and snuggle down into my mum's duvet. I can smell her perfume on the pillow and my eyes start to well up. It's only the second time I've cried this morning so I just brush the tears away and pretend no-one is there but me.

Soon I'm asleep and whether Demi is or not; she's lying there quietly, listening, learning; beginning to understand me, like no-one else does.

*****

Where's my memory gone? I don't have any memories now. I lost them all when I had Demi.

I don't remember anything; the last thing I can see in my mind is my wedding, a moving video of our dance.

I remember the sadness I felt when my babies died, I remember the pain I felt when my body was violated; but I hardly remember anything else.

I was a child? I don't remember it. Not a single memory of my first fifteen years. I may as well not have lived them because it's like amnesia hides who I was.

I like to listen to other people's stories of my life. Hear who I was from their words.

Because now I'm a different person; a new one. Someone I don't know yet.

*****

I'm sitting at the sea front with my Dad.
We're both quiet as Demi's asleep in the back.
When we're here we don't even need to speak.

It's a beautiful day; boiling hot and we are both baking; sweating in the heat.
If I look out my car window I can see my Dad's old house; his Gran-Grans house.
I know he's looking at it too; his eyes fixed on the upstairs window; the house that brought him joy every summer throughout his childhood.
And beyond it; beside that house; we can see Hengistbury Head; my Dad's Hengistbury Head.

"That should have been my house...." He says; the pain he's feeling inside, seeping through so that I am grieving for a woman and a home I never knew.
And I find myself nodding in agreement, because I've heard the story a thousand times. How his Gran-Gran wanted the house for him, and his family, and how his father stole it away from him, selling it, keeping the money for himself.
My Dad didn't even want the money. He didn't want it because it's a beautiful big house, he wanted it for the sentiment; the memories he holds, so that his Gran-Gran could live on....

And I see him looking at the water, scanning the sand, and he says "I'm looking for her. That's why I came back here; because it's as close as I can get to her. And I know I'll never find her, but I'll never, stop looking..."
And I see his face crumple, and the sadness creep into his eyes, darkening them on this beautiful day.

And I'm angry too. Angry at the Grandfather that used to buy me hundreds of toys and shower me with gifts and money, and I think about how as a child, I understood nothing, and now I know it all, and I wish I could have turned myself away from them, told him at eight years old that I didn't want those toys, I wanted my Dad to smile, and sit in his bedroom, the one he shared with his Gran-Gran and look out through the window with him to the ocean outside, so he could live forever, in the memories of a boy.

So we're sitting there silently, staring at this house, that's withered like a flower with no care. The sun doesn't shine on it the way it did when he was there.
I never knew it; I never lived it, and yet my mind sees it all.
I see him there as a child, sitting with his Gran-Gran, smiling and happy, away from the city life in Coventry, away from the boy he was there. I see him eating from posh China plates and walking along the Head with her hand in hand.
I know he grieves for her like one day I will grieve for him.

And he tells me how his heart is broken, for the way they

hurt her, and changed what could have been.

And I visualise the pain he felt, sitting at Christchurch station, waving goodbye to her, his heart splitting in his chest, but not crying; because big boys don't cry.

He sits beside me now, an old man, not too far from death, and my own heart starts to weep.

Because he holds these memories, the good times and the sad times and he keeps them all hidden inside, except for when he's with me, and that's when he opens up, and shares his life as a boy, coming to Bournemouth for his summer holidays; united with the only woman he has ever loved like that, only to be torn apart, dragged away from her at the end of the fun, leaving her behind, leaving the beauty and the freedom and the life he wishes he could live alongside her.

Back to Coventry and the shelters, the war and the poverty, and he sits on the train, proudly, like the man he wants to become, for her, and he glances out the window, and sees the Head in the distance, and there's the final stab, the last turn of the knife in his stomach, grinding the happiness away for another year.

So we sit and we look, at what was and what could have been, and I can almost hear his soul crying out to her, and I think about my babies in the ocean, and imagine her looking out through that top window, looking for my Daddy swimming fourteen lengths between the groins and watching over my babies I have placed just beside her.

*****

"I don't want to make them, I'm not doing it!" I'm shouting at Dino from the bedroom.
He's just come home from work and Demi is screaming for her bottle. There aren't any made and I can't bear the thought of doing them.

He's cross because he's tired and wants to sit down and rest.
"You're tired?? I'm fucking tired!!" I shout back.
"You've had all day long to wash them up..." I can hear him saying through gritted teeth.
"I don't care. I just couldn't do it." He doesn't understand. He probably thinks I'm lazy.
I couldn't muster the strength to go downstairs; I physically couldn't cope with the thought of making them.

He comes upstairs now with the baby and some milk.
She's still crying and I'm screaming for her to shut up and Dino just looks at me and shakes his head.
He lies her down with her bottle and immediately she's quiet.
I sigh and suddenly the room is silent, apart from the sound of her glugging from the bottle.

Dino's head is in his hands and I can hear him breathing deeply.
I want to breathe that calmly. My breath seems to be rapid and short.
I wish I could inhale as much oxygen as he can; let it fix my brain.
It's like the thought of having to make the bottles makes

me angry and miserable.

I don't want to make them; just like I don't want to wash my hair.
I can't even remember the last time I did.
It's greasy and heavy on my head. I know it needs to be clean; I want it to shine and be light like it was before I had her, but now it's smelly and ugly, and I think it needs to stay like that, because that's how I have to be now.
Dino and his Dad keep telling me how much weight I'm losing and it makes me feel sick just thinking about it.

I don't want to eat; I need to starve my body.
It's like when I'm chewing, my insides are angry.
I can feel my stomach growling, like it's shouting at me; hissing at me to feed it. But I'm angry; because my tummy is just a part of my insides; and now I hate every organ and every part of my body.
I can not stand the sight of myself.

Dino's telling me I'm beautiful, and I just hate him for even thinking it.
This being inside me, this thing that is taking me over, it tells me every day how hideous I am. I used to try and ignore it; push its violent voice away, but I can't anymore.
I'm forced to listen to it; believe it.

I can't even look at my own reflection. I had to take down all the mirrors last week. I'm still made to look at myself in the bathroom; I can't take his Dads mirror down. I just avoid it.

If I catch myself looking, just brush past it, I can feel my breath catch in my throat, like I'm suffocating on my own tongue and my heart starts to race.

I have to go back to bed then, and hide under the covers so I can't even find myself.

So now we're both just sitting here, silently.

I know he's probably angry at me; he's decided I've turned into a nasty person. I have.

I'm angry that the baby's quiet now. Always quiet when Dino's here; always happy then.

I think I've shot her an evil stare because Dino is watching me, his eyes wide with disbelief.

"WHAT?!" I scream waving my arms in the air like I've just been slapped.

He stands up and scoops her up in his arms.

"We'll be downstairs Rachel, come down when you've sorted yourself out....." and he's gone.

I can feel my face tighten and my chest rise and fall so quickly. I think I'm going to be sick. I'm so angry.

How dare he speak to me like that?? It's not my fault she doesn't love me; like me even.

"It's not my fault!" I'm shouting and sobbing now and before I know it, I've thrown her box across the room to the door.

Her beautiful box I spent so long preparing before she was born.

And it's bashed the wall and the corner is bent and now I'm even angrier and sadder and I can hear him coming back up the stairs.

I hide under the covers like a child and cry into my pillow.

I can hear him picking it up and moving towards me.

In my head I'm begging him to hold me tight and make me feel better.

My mind is screaming please Dino, please hold me and don't ever let me go.

But it doesn't work like that. My mind and my voice don't combine anymore. Now they collide; like they are enemies.

"Get off me!" I'm yelling. "Don't touch me!"

He knows I don't mean it though. He knows my lips speak something different to my mind, and he's just hugging me tighter through the thick covers.

And suddenly it dawns on me; he's left her downstairs. She's not crying, but he's with me and not with her, and suddenly I realise it's happened again, where I can't stand for him to be with her instead of me.

He's holding the covers tight around me and all I can think about is him pushing them onto my face so I can't breathe and won't have to suffer this anymore.

I'm shaking my head now because I hate these thoughts so much.

I don't hate her, do I? I love her right, I'm meant to love her!

Do I still love him, or do I despise him now, like sometimes I think I do?

I'm bashing my head up and down on the bed and I'm forcing myself not to cry, because the tears make me even angrier and constantly remind me, and him, that I'm not normal anymore.

*****

I'm playing cards with my Dad. The only game we ever play; trumps. Knock out whist it's called. I think he used to play it with his Gran-Gran. Games they enjoyed in the cooler days of the summer. Sitting sipping tea from beautifully decorated cups and saucers, nibbling biscuits he couldn't get enough of.

And we don't need to talk throughout this game. The deck and the hands we are dealt say all that needs to be said.
These games drag me away for a while. Separate my mind from how destroyed it's becoming.

He glugs the tea I've made him. No posh cups now, just a mug with best Dad scrawled on it; no biscuits.
And he beats me this time.
"Three - one..." He mutters amidst a fake cough. And I can't help but smile. 'Cause he's right. It's not my day today.

Then he's talking, his mind has wandered, and he's telling me about his first wife, about the amazing cakes she made him. That I'd never eat a cake like it, and I believe him, I believe every thing he tells me; I hang on every word.
And I know he loves her, I know a part of his heart belongs to her, and his other children, the babies he left so long ago.

And suddenly I see into his past again, his words describe everything.
How he walked out the door, pushing aside the sound of his daughter crying and begging him to stay and how his body felt tight with guilt and how his heart cried inside him.

His eyes look swollen, the colour seems to fade and his pupils take over, like reliving it still hurts him.
But when he talks to me, when he tells me how it was, it's like I listen like no-one else can.
I wasn't there to judge him; to see the truth. So I live my life, supporting him and loving him like no-one else can.

Because to me he is untouchable; unfaultable. My Daddy never sinned, my Daddy never wanted to hurt a soul, least of all his three babies. But it's only now as I'm growing, as I see things from an adults perspective, now that I see what did happen, who did get hurt, who was left to cope and cry alone, and I feel sad for all of them, but more for him, because that's how it shall always be; him and I united as one whole.

*****

How on earth can I explain it?? Don't touch me.
It's not that I don't love you, just please don't come near me.

Put the light on; quick. Oh my God I'm suffocating; I'm bleeding to death; someone is tearing me apart between my legs.

I'm hyperventilating....oh thank God, the light... I can see....no-one is here, no-one is hurting me.

Thank you for holding me. I don't think I ever thanked you.

No-one can hurt me when I'm in your arms.
I'm so embarrassed; I've ruined it...again.
I used to love to be with you; feel you touching and caressing me. But now I don't. It terrifies me. My skin goes prickly, but not in a good way anymore.
It's so sore....I'm trying to just think of you; but it keeps happening. I don't want to think about it, I'm not trying to remember it, just suddenly it's there in my mind every time you're stroking me.
I have to try again; I don't want this. I'm going to force it out of my mind.
It's fine. I'm ok. It feels good.....then why are my legs forcing you away, you ask?? Oh God.

I am screaming in my head for them to stop it I swear. I want you inside me again. I promise.
I'm so rigid I could be dead. My body is stiff as stone, I know it.
You keep asking me if I'm ok. I know you care; you'd never force me like they did.
I can't though. And now I'm sobbing.

I hate this, I hate it so much I want to scream and gauge my own face apart.
This never used to happen. I never used to have to think

59

about it. I never even remembered it.
Now it's here to haunt me.

*****

*I'm a zombie today. I see through eyes of stone, sadness. I do
not live or feel; I just am.
I wake and I sleep. I wake and then sleep again. I take
my pills in a mild awakeness.. Drift in and out of reality,
slowly fade away from humanity. In to the black world,
that I begin to desire.
I sit as if paralysed. My limbs move, in utter understanding
and of purpose. Yet my soul feels motionless. Glued to my
insides.
I hear her and I see her tears, yet there's no emotion. I see
him and I hold him, yet I am not myself today.
Behind my dusty eyes of emptiness I feel hollow and sick
inside.
Where has my person gone; the being I once was?
When will she return?*

*****

It's Friday today and this is my new favourite day of the
week. The doctor said I need something to look forward
to. This is definitely it.

Dino will be home soon and I'm packing Demi's little
pink bag for Dad.
I keep smiling today; I feel light inside, like I'm floating
on a cloud.
No-one's going to upset me today; everyone knows this
is my good day.

Dino's home and I think I've hugged him already.

He's bought me a bottle of WKD; not that I need it to help me sleep.

God I can't wait for the pillow. I know the second my head hits it, I'll be gone.

No nightmares tonight; I don't get them on a Friday.

I don't need to keep getting up; I don't need to watch her sleep tonight. Or listen for her breathing, Daddy will do that for me.

All her bottles are made. I can't remember when I did them; it must be magic on a Friday.


Soon enough we're alone.

I don't feel sad about leaving her there. She's used to it.

She has her beautiful Australian crib there. I think she likes it more than her Moses basket at our house.

Dad sits and swings her; sings her to sleep like I can't.

I know she loves him more than she loves me.

I think she should be with him every night.

I'm sitting on the bed; smiling I think.

Tonight's a good night.


Dino puts my programme on and I can't wait for it to start. He's made me a nice supper and he's cosying up next to me.

I have a few sips of my drink and already I can feel myself relax.

I know Dino's smiling inside.


Now I don't have to be this evil person. The evil's gone for the night.

It does when I'm not with Demi. Funny that.
My mind doesn't really wander much. I don't need to worry about her; she's with him; safe like she should be.

*****

Monday. That means Dino's back at work and I have all week to wait for my next night of peace from the baby and the pain.
I hate this day; I hate every single day of the week now.
Apart from Friday. That's the day I love; my happy day.
I need to go to my parents when Dino is home. We all need to go there so I can smile for a while.

Dino will put Demi in the car.
I refuse to do her seat.
It doesn't dawn on me for a long time why.
I think I hated doing anything that would benefit her.
I couldn't bathe her, I couldn't do her nappy, I couldn't feed her, and I couldn't strap her in so she was safe.
Like I was leaving the gaps; allowing something to hurt her.
I didn't hurt her. I thought about it a lot though.
Thoughts I never want to share; not with anyone.

So instead of doing it; instead of tearing her up inside the way I was, I just left the spaces; not protecting her like I should have been.
That still haunts me now.

*****

Suddenly the sky is dark and there's rain.

Now it changes; the anger and pain soften, and now I'm filled with the same terror I get every day when I'm alone with her.

That man again; the same man that always haunts me since having her.

Since the memory came back.

He's coming for us. Not just me this time; her too. He's angry with me for remembering; for knowing.

I've made sure the door is locked, but it doesn't matter. He can get through locked doors; walls even. This man is amazing.

Nothing can stop him.

So now all I can do is wait.

I shut us in the bedroom upstairs. Dino didn't put a lock on the inside of the bedroom door like I'd asked. He was probably afraid I'd try to kill myself.

But now I want it; I need the barrier, just in case his powers have faded and I can block him out.

So now the drawers are there.

I've used so much energy putting them there. I had to lie her down in her cot and drag them inch by inch. I think I took too many iron tablets but I needed the strength; like they make my blood thicken and ooze.

I have to draw the curtains so he can't see in; see me shaking with fear.

The vent on the wall is covered with her picture.

I can't let him see through it; spying on us. I need to put her picture there, so every time I glance at it, she reminds me of why we need to hide.

I can hear the door open. My breathing seems to have stopped.

She's looking up at me with her eyes wide, like she knows; she heard it to.

I'm not imagining it.

I can hear the lock turn behind him. He must have gotten a spare. I knew it.

Now he's on the stairs, I can hear every step he takes. It's like the floor boards are echoing what's coming.

She starts crying and it's like all my senses are back, tripling the effect of every sound.

And I've scooped her up; I'm cradling her now, drawing her into my chest.

Anything to shut her up.

He'll hear you, I'm whispering to her.

I'm begging her to be quiet and I'm hiding under my dressing gown.

My eyes are stinging; I'm forcing the tears to disappear. I'm not going to cry; I'm not going to let him see me cry.

I've never held her so tight before.

I don't want him to hurt her.

In a matter of seconds my mind has foretold me my death. I know how he's going to stab me in the neck. Repeat my old nightmare.

All the while she'll watch, she will sit there and watch me scream and writhe with the agony of it all. She'll watch me die and then, when I'm not there to protect her, then he'll do it to her.

She's quiet now, and so am I.

"Rachel? Hello?" It's Dinos Dad.

I'm too stunned at first to speak.

"Oh Hi!" I manage to shout back through the barricaded door.

He mutters something about running a bath and making his dinner and I just sit there in disbelief.

My whole body goes limp, like it needs to relax. Every muscle aches from the strength I'd used.

I look at the baby and shake my head.

She stares back up at me, happy now; rubbing her eyes, like she's tired, like none of it even affected her.

I put her back in to her cot and try to silently move the furniture back; because I don't need the door blocked anymore. I don't need the protection when someone else is there.

He'd never come when I'm not alone.

It's only solitude that invites him.

\*\*\*\*\*

*Dino's written in my diary:*
*I just want to hold you*
*She won't even talk to me; she won't even look at me,*
*She's trying to push me away.*
*Every day I'm finding it harder and harder to resist and I*
*think should I just let her*
*push me away?*
*But I don't want this.*
*Why would she do this?*
*I love her.*

*What have I done to make her feel this way?*
*It tears me apart to see her like this,*
*I want to help but she is making it so hard.*
*If she wanted help then why would she push the people she*
*loves away?*
*Let me love you.*
*I don't want to be pushed away.*
*I just want to hold you and let you know I care.*


\*\*\*\*\*


I'm so angry today. I wanted to go out for dinner with Dino and the baby but we don't have any money and I'm in a really bad mood. Dino is offering to cook us dinner but I can't even look at him.

"I don't want any. Go away!" I'm acting like a spoilt child. I can't have my own way so I'm taking it out on him like I always do.
"You're hungry Rachel you need to eat here..." He is insisting I have some dinner here but I'm refusing and turning away from him, scowling and pouting. Thinking of the days I used to love cooking meals for him.

I have to go upstairs and get away from the smell of the oven and the sausages frying in the pan. I used to love his dinners, homemade comfort food as Mum and he call it. Now I can't even bear to think of it.
My stomach hurts where I haven't eaten again today. I know I'll wake up in the middle of the night though and scoff as much chocolate as I can find while Dino's asleep.
Like I don't want him to ever see me eat again. Not in the

house anyway.

I don't want him to see me chewing and swallowing mouthfuls of food, so now I need to do it in secret or distract myself if someone's in the room, staring at me eating. Sometimes it feels like slow motion, like every time my jaw meets to crush the meat the sound of it is deafening and people are going to be sick all around me.

So today I sit and sulk, spend my evening alone, avoiding him, not talking to him, blaming him for the way I'm feeling and I starve myself until two in the morning when I feed Demi her milk and sit in the dark, huddled under the covers so no-one can see my ugly body, while I feed it squares of chocolate and lumps of cakes I don't even like.

And then I'm cutting my leg again; angry at the lumps of fat squelching beneath my skin; furious with myself for eating, ashamed of myself for not being able to have just starved and not given in to the aching hollowness that my stomach has become.

So now I trace the blade along my inner thigh, piercing the skin again, relaxing at the feeling that takes over my body, releasing the pain, reminding me that I'm alive.

My mind is constantly telling me to punish myself for being so fat and ugly; incapable and weak. Like slicing at such a soft area of flesh makes my body feel so fragile and precious; convincing me not to kill myself, not to cut too deep, just to see how much I can take without passing out, how much this new feeling can help me let go of all these vicious feelings and thoughts inside.

*****

I need to be by the sea again; I need to be close to my babies, like when we're united, it's a force far stronger than any other and the evil is bundled away; broken.
I've begged him to bring me again. He tuts, because when he sees the water, his heart aches too.

We can see a little boat in the distance; not far from the horizon.
Dad wishes he'd had a boat; could have floated away in the sunshine.

In my mind I can see that.
Him as a young lad, with his Gran-Gran sitting beside him, in her elegant tweed suit; her wavy golden hair floating in the breeze.

I begin to wonder if I'll forever grieve for this woman. This lady that my father loved so very much; that I never met and never knew.

Pain pierces me as I see his stare drift off and I know he's remembering; reliving the Christmases he shared with her as a boy and I wish so much I could bring it all back for him; just for a moment so he could see her; hold her.
And he tells me how he remembers swimming in the water; the very same water we are looking at now, fifty years on, and how his tummy scraped the sand below and how he loved to swim; and I think back to when I placed my babies there; how when he was just a child he never knew what his life would bring, or that I'd place the babies I had lost right with him; with the soul of the

boy he was.

I feel ok now, because I know I have some money so tonight I'll get to eat and can fill my mouth with scampi and vegetables, brought out to me on a nice clean plate; it's preparation not even on my mind.

But as I finish, I notice people staring at me, looking right at me, appalled by the state of me. I'm wearing my Dads baggy t-shirt, desperate to hide what's underneath, and my hair is hardly brushed.
I'm in trousers that are loose around my thighs and I've got yesterdays make-up stained around my eyes.
Dino doesn't say anything, he would never say anything mean to me, but I don't even need him to because all the eyes are following me now.

I need to get out of here. I've shovelled the last mouthful in and I'm standing already. Dino's looking up at me, half his pint sitting untouched and he says he needs to let his stomach settle and finish his beer, but I can't wait that long; so now I'm dashing, swerving past the people around me, staring at the ground, trying not to breathe, just get past them and out into the open air so that I can breathe again, where no-one knows I've just eaten and so I can get home and hide where no-body has to look at me.

*The sun shines no more, just dark deep shadows covering*

*the light.*
*Fears enclosed hairs on end, shivers down my spine.*
*Tears build up in my eyes, but I'm determined not to let*
*them flow.*
*My cheeks, cold, freeze my fingers as I touch my skin,*
*intending to warm myself up.*
*The shadows at the edges of the trees, move in the wind as*
*the leaves blow.*
*Wind gushes all about, I never realised how loud it could*
*be.*
*Faint sounds I recognise as screams, spirits all around me,*
*I'm sure they're here.*
*Leaves blow off the trees and float past me, brushing at my*
*side, ticking my cheeks,*
*startling me.*
*I try and smile, thinking how close to home I am,*
*But I forget it as soon as I hear the sounds again.*
*They spin all around me, everywhere I turn, I hear them.*
*They fill my head with evil, I hear them speak,*
*Words I never heard anyone say before, a new language I*
*can understand.*
*My mind is confused, I hear words but there is no-one there*
*to speak them.*
*I begin to shake now, I'm so scared and frightened, and so*
*alone. I wish I wasn't*
*alone.*
*It's so dark and so quiet, beside the voices I just can't shake*
*off.*
*I hear only their cries and their pain.*
*I can't help them, as hard as I try, I can't.*
*Their voices, their screams and shouts, drown out the rest of*
*what I hear.*

*I cry now.*
*I'd tried so hard to resist the tears, but now there is no hope.*
*The salty tears trickle down my cheeks, burning them as they go.*
*I spin about, try and block out the sounds, but it's hopeless and in the end I give up.*
*I cry and cry until I can cry no more.*
*I fall to the ground, all is lost, and the voices will never leave.*

\*\*\*\*\*

Why does she have to refer to it as a mental illness? Why does she have to keep saying that? Using those words that feel like they're ripping at my brain and shredding it to pieces!

It's making me angry, like I can feel my heart start to race again and my blood boil inside me. I want to scream at her to leave me alone; to get the hell away from me because the last thing I need right now is her down my throat banging on about how crazy I'm going.

I wish I could fade away....sometimes I wish the evil man that wants me would just take me away so I don't have to feel any pain anymore....but I know that's crazy in itself, because if he got hold of me, he'd torture me and severe my limbs like I see him do in my nightmares.

# July 2006

We're packed and ready to go. I've never been so excited. It's out first year in Cornwall as a 'family' and I can't wait to be there.

The coach trip is hard as it gives me plenty of time to think and I can feel myself getting anxious again so I try and focus on something else and I watch the trees and animals as we drive by, wondering if the ewe's feel this shitty when they have their lambs.

Soon we're there though and I can't get through the front door fast enough. I can't stop smiling and I just run up the stairs, beckoning Dino to bring the baby so I can show her the bedroom I've been sleeping in each summer since I was nine.

I think I'm jumping on the bed, maybe rolling all over it and Dino can't stop smiling and he looks so happy and I can see Demi kicking her legs in her chair. And then I run out of energy and Dino asks me if I've taken an iron tablet today and then it hits me and the crash begins and my smile fades and my body starts working over time to try and pump what little blood I have around my brain and my limbs and then I'm crying, and I don't even know why, and Dino's arms are round me once more, holding me, squeezing me into him, like he always does, and still, she is watching; always watching.

*****

We've been here three days and already my bright mood has died. I'm sitting on the bed I sat on twelve years ago, but now I'm an adult, though it feels inside like I still want cuddling and rocking. I've got the knife in my hand and I'm drawing
patterns on my thighs. It feels exciting to see the little white lines I'm tracing cover my legs, but it's just the beginning.
That's not the release I need. I poke the tip harder, until I feel it pierce and then I lightly drag the blade along my thigh.

Suddenly I can hear someone coming; him most probably and I have to shove the knife under the duvet and cover my leg quickly.
"You ok babe?" He asks me, sitting himself down, almost right beside the hidden knife. I smile and nod at him and pretend to be concentrating on my book.
I want him to go away so we don't have to row and I don't need to shout or cry; I just want him to go so I can carry on making myself feel better. I think he knows something is wrong though; he always knows; sometimes I forget how well he understands me.

So I have to start shouting at him. He's trying to comfort me. He asks if I've had my anti-depressants and I use that as ammunition to scream at him to get out. That how I feel has nothing to do with those stupid pills and that I don't even need them.

I know he wants me to calm down, but how can I get better if I have to accept what is happening. That the evil is taking over my body and my mind.

Eventually I can see that I've hurt him and he leaves the room, probably has to feed the baby by now. Then I start getting angry, stupid damn baby needs feeding right when I need him to be with me. Then I'm even angrier. I don't care if she needs

feeding, I don't want him up here anyway. Plus, if he doesn't feed her, she can just keep crying, 'cause I'm not doing it, I can't stand to go near her when she's crying like that.

And soon, I am sobbing; crying uncontrollably. I know the thoughts I'm having; I'm so terrified someone else can read my mind.

I just want my Dino back; I just want my baby and me to be ok.

But we're not damnit, are we?! What the hell is wrong with me?!

Then I'm practically screaming and throwing myself around the room, and soon he's there again, with his arms around me, crying too, holding me still so I can't hurt myself anymore. And I think he's seen the knife, or my legs, or whatever, but I feel ashamed and dirty and now I'm scarred, so I'll never forget what I'm doing.

"I have to punish myself" I'm sobbing as he's rocking me.

"I need to stop the pain in my heart.....I need to die

now..." and I'm trailing off 'cause I can't keep focused and my body's giving way so he lies me down on the bed and I think he's swaying me to put me to sleep 'cause by now he knows I can't do it
by myself anymore.

And I'm thinking about what I've done, and I'm thinking what he's doing for me, and I know he's going back down to her in a minute and I thank God he's so much stronger than I am and that he can look after the baby that most days I can't even bear to look at.

So I ask him, through my half asleep state, "No-one can see it can they? You've done her buttons up, right?" and he knows exactly what I'm talking about because he understands my obsession with it, so he smoothes back my hair and reassures me that no-one can see her cyst and that she's fine now she's got her milk and that she loves her mummy for wanting to protect her, and I don't know whether to scream or sob, so I just do nothing, and I wait for sleep to rescue me.

*****

I'm sitting in the bedroom, staring at the flowery wallpaper that I've stared at since I was a small child.
The spare cot is pushed up against the wall and I'm tracing the embossed design with my finger; the beautiful pinks and greens drawing me in to their swirls, saving my mind.

And soon the blanket is to my chest. The gorgeous quilt they've placed in the old cot for my baby. Its pink fluffy cotton pulled in to me; soothing me, comforting me like a baby.

I can hear Mum's music downstairs, the sheep bleating from the field, the rain pitter pattering on the glass beside me; heavy droplets in a musical pattern.

I'm closing my eyes; trying to focus on my body and my mind as one again.

I'm so confused; my mind is so very fuzzy and I try to remember the person I used to be. The child I was when we first came here; loud, bubbly, happy.

I decide if I lie here for long enough, that little girl will creep from the bed sheets back in to my body.

*****

We're home again. Not our home; not our flat; my parent's house; my home.

I miss them; I wish my parents could come back early too.

Dino's at work and I can't bear it.

I love it here. I need to be here 24/7. When I'm with my Daddy the evil subsides.

It knows it can't get me when I'm in his presence. He's too strong for it; I wish I was that strong.

I need to go back; we need to go back to Cornwall.

Dino tries to reassure me they'll be back soon.

We're sitting in their bed. I need to sleep in their bed to be as close as possible to them; breathe in their smells, my Mums perfume stained on her pillow.

"We're looking after the house right Rach? They need some space babe..." I'm trying to block out what he's saying.

"You don't understand Dino..." He doesn't get it. He doesn't know that when I'm with my Daddy the sadness lifts if even only slightly.

*****

Dino's written in my diary again:

*Hi Princess,*

*How are you? You looked beautiful tonight. I really enjoy doing things with you right now, even if we just go for a walk.*

*I'm sorry I can't make you happy. And go back to Cornwall. I would love to take you back there you know that, don't you?*

*I'm sorry you're finding things so hard with Demi right now.*

*I'm sorry that you might not be going back to work and seeing Cody.*

*You wrote before in here, 'I want to be with my baby, but I want to be with my Cody too; he needs me so much.'*

*I know you love him Poppet, but Demi also needs you.*

*More so, you're her Mother and she needs you to be there for her.*

*These are important years and spending time with Demi will help you bond together.*

*You're a wonderful wife Rachel. You mean the world to me and I love you so much and always will.*

*Dino x x*

*****

I glance at the wood on the wall, framing the poem

77

I wrote him years ago; a picture beside it, of him and I a decade ago. And now I miss him more than ever; like him being two hundred miles away withdraws him completely from my life.

I think I'm crying again; pushing the baby away and Dino's sighing and speechless again and he tells me we can go, and then it's happened; I'm transformed already. I'm so excited. I have to tell Mum. I can't wait.

I can pack again; I can get her away from this; away from me.

*****

We all come back together; like it should be. Home on the same day.

I still can't go though; so I'm begging everyone to let us stay.

"We'll go in the spare room Mum; it's just for one night. I can't bear to go home!" And before I know it; everyone's setting the room up. Demi's travel cot is up and my bag is unpacked on the floor and I'm safe again.

It feels so right here.

I'm sitting on the spare bed, looking at the empty room, loving that none of my meaningless belongings are here to cloud my mind and the beautiful clarity of the room.

I don't think Dino gets it. He wants to go back to our lovely new flat. I know he loves it there but I don't ever want to leave here again.

*****

I'm walking around in a daze. I feel trapped up here; in

our claustrophobic flat.

I can't get used to it. Now I hate it like I hated our last home.

I'm right at the top. I have to close all the sloping windows; not let any light in.

I'm swamped with solitude again.

Dad and Dino tell me to keep myself busy; not let the bad thoughts intrude.

So I look around the flat; move slowly from each room. Stare at what needs to be done; the washing up, the dirty laundry, the state of the grubby carpets, but it all seems too much, it feels like this tiny home is crushing me; closing in around me.

I walk to my calendar and check I've had my pills each day and I study the dosage and wonder if having more will make things better.

Demi sleeps in her room, the one I decorated to look so pretty, and I sit here alone in the dark, feeling so desperately lonely and yet too afraid to leave.

So I light a cigarette in my own company.

I know Dino will know; he'll smell it on me and hate me for it; like I've taken drugs or something.

And then I'm inhaling, and it's the closest I can get back to the gas and air that saved me before from all the pain.

I'm dizzy and my head is spinning and I feel the toxins poison my insides like he says they will.

And I'm lying on the floor, eyes closed, head swirling, like a cigarette has given me the feelings of a drug like an ecstasy pill and the thought crosses my mind because this feeling isn't too great, but it's distracting me. And I'm sucking on the tip, drawing all the toxins into my mouth; certain that I need the poison inside me, that it's meant just for me, to destroy the body I'm forced to live within; kill the lungs that cruelly make me breathe and feel this pain. My legs are shaking and I'm watching the tobacco burn and turn to ash; like I'm inhaling its evil and I know it's destroying me inside. The nicotine filling my blood and my veins; helping me cope, like now the only way I can survive is to focus on the evil and surrender to it.

Soon she is crying and I have to crawl to her room, trying not to vomit on the way, lying on the carpet beside her cot, curled up, and talking to her through the wooden bars. Trying to focus on her but failing miserably as my mind descents into the darkness again.

*****

I'm at the Head; Hengistbury Head. I'm walking up the long slope and I'm pushing my heavy body against the wind that's trying to force me away again.
I must get to the top; I need to be up there; as high as I can be; close to the souls of the ones I love.

And then I'm there; kneeling in the dry soil, fingering the twigs on the ground, stroking their stems, twisting them between my fingers. Thinking of the life they live, the air the leaves breathe; the same air that gives me life.

The green shoots are poking through their broken skin and their sap is leaking like my blood, swimming out of me where the sharp edge of the silver blade presses into my pores and my feeble flesh; so fragile and lean.

*****

It's Friday again, and I'm safe from the evil for now.
I can't bear us to be here for a night alone.
We need to sleep at my parents' house tonight. A spare mattress in the lounge is all I need.

Dino's got my WKD like it's a ritual. I don't need anything stronger now. I don't need the shots or the spirits tonight.
All I need is the freedom from the hatred inside me.
I pop upstairs and see my Dad, sitting on the edge of his bed; Demi's in the crib, asleep already. How does he do it, why does it take me hours and hours to calm her?
I know she's safe now, safe in his presence, like I am downstairs.

And Jo and Skip are here; sleeping on the cushions beside us, and I feel so happy now; so normal.
We all watch the tele and snack and laugh and it feels so good to be with the people I love most and know I have Demi, but have her upstairs, so I don't need to look at her and be constantly reminded of what I've become.

I realise today that I love Skip, love him as my brother, not just a normal brother-in-law. He's my family for good now. He's my husbands little brother, my little sisters partner, the father of my nephews, and today I see him like I've not seen him before, like it doesn't matter anymore that it was he that put me in to early labour, that he fills his days with deliberately irritating me, none of it even matters, what matters is that when I need them, they are here, and I just know now that he will always be here for me, no matter what. Loving me in return as a real sister.

And Jo. My precious little sister Joanna.
It is her that dries my tears during the week, the days I'm forced to deal with what is happening to me, her that comforts Demi when I'm not able to. When she cries from the colic and my brain is screaming in my head to just damn well shut her up; it is Jo that takes her, rocks her, talks to her like I can't.
And I just want to hold her, cradle my baby sister, the girl that shared the moment with me, the moment I'm forced to always remember, where she stabbed at the insides of me with her intruding unwelcome fingers.

***** 

It's the weekend and Dino's downstairs with my Dad and the baby. I'm lying in my Mums bed, curled up and hiding. I told her I didn't want to go shopping anymore and she's come upstairs, bursting in to the room, plonking herself down beside me and pulling the covers back from my face.
She can see the tears leaking from my eyes; tuts and turns away.

"For God sake Rachel, pull yourself together, you've got everything you want. Get up and get over it!" and with that she is gone and I'm left alone again, in shock and paralysed with the pain inside.

Now my tears are falling faster and heavier and my chest hurts inside, 'cause I can still smell her perfume and hear her words ringing in my head.

"Get over it. Get over it. Get over it." And all I want to do is die right now, because I know she is right, I know I have everything I could ever have wanted, I know I've got the baby I so desperately craved, but I can't help it, I don't know what's wrong with me, I don't understand why I feel this way and then I am doing it again, using all I can find, a nail file hiding in her drawer and I'm punishing myself again for feeling this way and not being able to just jump up and 'get over it' like she wants me to.

She doesn't understand at all. I think it's so hard for her because she's such a strong person. She can control her emotions.

She never let what happened to her bring her down. She isn't weak like I am; she wouldn't let it poison her the way it poisons me inside and I am so ashamed of myself. I wish I could make her love me again; understand what's wrong with me, but I can't, so now I'm forced to push her away; hide what's really going on in my mind and cut the love I have for her and the way I need my Mummy more than ever.

*****

*I'm dreaming again; of the man that used to be...*
*One time in the dark of the night,*
*You spun round and gave me a fright.*
*You looked at me bitterly, spoke to me brittley,*
*And told me you wanted me to die.*
*Three years of my life I gave you,*

*A ring on my finger,*
*I kept from you, the scars on my arms,*
*A memory of the love, from you.*
*You'd never done anything like this before,*
*You just kept frightening me, more and more.*
*I tried to resist you, turn from the pain,*
*But you kept on puncturing me,*
*Leaving red blood stains.*
*I held my breath, afraid to move,*
*Scared you were still there, trying to prove, your control.*
*You didn't stop though, your mind power driven,*
*You kept on kicking, pushing the position.*
*I could taste my own blood, wet to my lips,*
*Listening to you shouting, fearful for the kids.*
*It was then I heard him cry, my only pride and joy,*
*And I knew that you would stop,*
*Pick him up and drop, him down beside me.*

It's just a dream, it's just a dream; it's just a dream.

# August 2006

Now I'm back in their bedroom. The baby on my lap; crying with the colic, struggling against my cuddles. And the tears are falling; drowning my face with their weight.
I've got the tiny lamp on beside me, like it always is when we are up here.
The bright light hurts my eyes but I need enough to keep me from the blackness.
I can't soothe her anymore; I can't comfort her endlessly without success.

Then Jo is in the room, suddenly beside me.
Taking the baby from me and bouncing her on her lap. She rocks her backwards and forwards, holding her right arm below her stomach, pushing on the pain in my daughters' body, and her other hand, her beautifully painted nails are stroking me, combing through my matted hair, relaxing me.
The silence is deafening, pounding in my head.
And I'm so grateful that she is here; stopping the awful noise that infuriates me when she cries.

But then I'm angry. I'm so angry and bitter than she stopped for her. I tried the same, but it doesn't work with me.

Like the baby knows I don't care, that I just want her to stop for my own sake; for the sanity of my own mind.

I close my eyes and pretend to sleep; if I look at her I'll scream.

She kisses my cheek and asks me if I'm ok, offers to take Demi downstairs so I can sleep.

Immediately I start shouting.

"I don't need your help. Just go away. You don't need to take my baby away. I don't need anybody's help!"

I'm staring at her, forcing my tears to subside. Piercing her with my eyes full of hatred, and I think she's stunned, believing me ungrateful, which is how I know I appear.

And then she is gone. And I'm alone again, in the dim lit room, with just the baby beside me.

Quiet now, she's served her purpose. I don't need her, or anyone.

And then my chest is rising and falling, my breathing quickening, because I'm so very angry.

I'm so angry at the baby, and at Jo for knowing I need help and I'm furious with myself for speaking to her like that; shouting at my baby sister; pushing her love and kindness away, and then the knife is out from hiding, drawing along my thigh, breaking the skin so easily; punishing me again for being so evil.

*****

I'm out drinking again. I'm going to get drunk, try and hide the dull ache inside me.

Dino's at home with the kids. He probably thinks I'm

going to cheat on him. He always thinks that. I've given up trying to make him believe I won't. He doesn't understand what I'm going through though. I don't want another man, Jesus, I can't even please the one I've got right now.

I'm not really enjoying myself. It's like when I go to bingo with Dino's sister. I don't even find it fun anymore. It just makes the hours go by, without being stuck, sat next to a baby that hates me and a husband that probably can't stand the sight of me anymore.
I'm downing the shot, not really aware of whether it's my fifth or sixth. Does it matter? I'm still a shit Mum. I look at the drinks behind the bar and ask for something stronger; maybe a shot will clear my mind...ha...ha...here goes.....nope, still a shit Mum, in fact, now an even worse Mum.

I puff on the cigarette I swore to Dino I wouldn't smoke. It tastes fowl, but it fills my lungs with a legal poison and right now I can't think of anything better.
My friends are laughing and joking. Part of me manages to smile alongside them, and just for a minute, I'm not a mummy anymore. I'm not a wife, I'm not depressed, and I don't have serious fucking problems.

But then after the seventh or eighth drink, I remember, that is my life. The Mummy bit isn't bad, and neither is the wife part, just the whole I wish I was dead thing that I can't seem to shift!

Some bloke tries to put his arm around me, but despite

being dizzy I just shrug him off and make my way outside.

I want to go home. I want to go to bed and lie next to Dino.

I'm suddenly stumbling through the door...the taxis gone, thank God; I don't know how much more small talk and false smiles I can manage.

I push the front door open, trying to be quiet. I don't want to wake them; I just want to watch them sleep so quietly and peacefully.

I walk past Demi's door, but I can't hear anything. I keep going to our room, and as soon as I nudge the door I can hear them.

Both of them snoring; it makes me smile.

She's come into our room and is snuggled up in his arms on the edge of the bed.

Now I'm in a heap on the floor, crying, shaking. I want them to be this happy all the time. Whenever I'm here they're not. I disrupt their happiness and stamp my foot on their smiles.

My throat is still warm from the sambuca, hot right down through my body, burning at the evil inside me.

I need to be part of them. I throw my clothes off and climb in beside him. I put my arms around him but I think he's had a few drinks himself and he's not waking up in a hurry.

For just a while I feel part of a family; a family who love each other; a happy family.

And then I sob once again, in his arms, tears that seem to

never stop coming.

I realise in my dizzy state that it's the fourth night I've left them this week. I feel sick inside, but funnily enough I don't think it's the alcohol. I am ashamed of myself; as a wife, and as a mother. I've let my family down and I don't understand why. I go to sleep crying, confused, wanting more from my life and for theirs.

*****

I can't change it though; I'm powerless to the desire I have inside to change. So I'm out at bingo again, wasting money I don't have, that my husband works long hours to provide for us, feeling alone and morbid and guilty, wanting to be beside him and hold her in my arms, cradling the baby I always wanted.

But the evil inside me is pushing those feelings away; blocking them out of my mind, telling me that if I go home to them, I'll just be worse, crying in their company, ruining them as well.

So I sit and frown, hating what I'm doing and who I'm with, listening as though the man calling the numbers is counting down to my death, like every digit I see flashing green in front of me will somehow kill me. And I use this opportunity to eat. Stuffing biscuits and chips in to my mouth while no-one else can see; like all the other people in this hall are invisible, and my husband and my baby won't know I've eaten, won't know that I'm feeding this wickedness inside me.

And then it's late and dark outside, and the light breeze is twirling in my hair, while I wait for the car and jump in beside them, speeding off down the roads, the adrenaline pumping inside me, reminding me again that I am alive and the body I live within is precious, however angry I am at it for inhabiting the evil that fills me with sin.

*****

*I can't socialise at the moment; I'm not in the mood. I don't want to talk to anyone. I don't even want to look at anyone's face.*
*I don't want to have to smile and make chit-chat. I don't want to parade around and pretend everything's ok.*
*I don't want to hear her announce that I am getting better. I'm sick of hearing her say that because she can't handle the truth.*
*It makes me so angry. I am so mad at her for not wanting to help me or understand me; but why should she? Why should she want to? Why should anybody want to?*
*I now have to go and smile and tell everyone I'm enjoying myself because if I don't I'll get accused of spoiling everybody's fun.*
*All I want to do though is curl up and hide away again. Turn away from all the smiles and cry alone.*

# October 2006

I'm back at work now. How hilarious. If people knew how I was feeling inside they'd probably do anything to get me away from this boy. I'm supposed to help him, and yet I think it's him who's helping me.

I missed him so much. I think right now I love him more than I love my own baby.

He's smiling at me and he asks about her. I don't want to talk about her for long though so I change the subject and try and get him to focus on his work.

I worked with children with Autism and Aspergers Syndrome for two years before I had Demi, including working with Cody here at a mainstream school for roughly six months.

Nothing else in life compares to when I'm with this boy. He's ten, well eleven now, but I missed his eleventh birthday as I was on maternity leave.

I'm back now though, and there's no where else I'd rather be.

Dad's got Demi, best place for her I imagine. And I'm back with my boy; the most wonderful boy in the world.

I'm not the same person anymore. I'm not miserable Rachel. I'm not Rachel with Post Natal Depression. I'm not Demi's Mum.

I'm Mrs. Day to Cody and there's no other way I want to be seen.

I don't need to hear his problems from his lips; I don't need him to tell me what's wrong or try and explain. I just know.

I'm shit at maths; I didn't excel in school; I don't have any special talents, but when I'm with these kids, I'm incredible.

There's a bond we share now, that I don't think either of us have with another person. He looks at me, and I understand everything that's going on in his mind and to a degree, I think he gets me too.

My baby should be enough to get me out of bed each morning, but the truth is, right now, it isn't. I'm pulling myself together each day for this boy, for this one child, that has never ever hurt me, that has never ever made me feel sad or angry or confused. It's him I want to spend every day with, it's him I want to help and talk to.

I like that he confides in me, I like that things piss him off, just the same as they do me, only he's got the balls to speak up,

although that's probably not how it's supposed to be seen!

I have to tell him that he needs to think about what he is saying, not to be rude, to use his manners etc....but really inside, I'm thinking, you're so brave Code, you're so opinionated and strong-minded. I admire him. I love him.

I don't feel depressed when I'm with him. I don't have any

anxiety problems. I don't get scared or angry or hurt. I just smile, the whole time. I feel strong and independent.

He makes me laugh and smile and every time he tries hard at his work, it makes me feel so proud. 'Cause I know he's doing it just for me. He's doing it 'cause I asked him to. He won't do it when they tell him to. He doesn't want to do what they say. But I just have to look at him, and let my soul touch his with my gaze and he lives up to the very, very high expectations I hold for him and makes me proud.

And then I'm struggling, and it's the only bad day I've had, 'cause a boy called me fat to his friends and I over heard him, and I know he's right and suddenly I feel like a bullied child and my tears are welling up and Cody and I are upstairs working on an English sheet, but I have to turn away and stare out the window as I remember how sharp it stabbed me in the chest.

But he knows you see. He can tell I'm sad and however adult or professional I try and be, he wants to know why I'm sad. So I find myself telling him. Though I think he already knew and he looks into my eyes and I just stare back. I'm an adult and here I am, opening up to an eleven year old child about one of his peers calling me fat and making me cry.

I want to shoot myself in the head for how unprofessional this is, but something stops me. I think it's his hand on mine. He just looks up at me with his beautiful eyes and tells me "You're not fat Mrs. Day you've just had a baby" and inside my chest is burning because I can't believe the empathy he has just shown me, when it's one of the things children with Aspergers often suffer with, and I can't believe this moment is even happening, so I thank him for his kindness and change the subject, but the truth is, I'll never forget this minute. It's stamped in my memory forever. Because I think he's amazing. I really, truly do.

And yet nobody knows the emotions I hide inside. Just like they don't know some days I want to take my own life.

I will never, ever forget him. I like to think I helped him through his last year at mainstream primary school, and that he helped me more than he or anybody else will ever know. He helped me deal with post-natal depression and to fall in love with my own daughter.

*****

I'm thinking of the boys I used to work with:
*He can speak no words, just communicate through sounds,*
*Noises that are true to him, words that reach no bounds.*
*Stares that see only emptiness, darkness in the light,*
*Cloudy bubbles shadow his eyes, blurring the real sight.*
*Whispers in his ears, imaginary sounds,*
*Blocking out the words I speak, the ones that reach no bounds.*
*If he does focus on me, and stare past all the clouds,*
*It's as if he looks right through me, to another black and white world.*
*Maybe he sees my lips moving, but lives in only silence,*
*Perhaps he hears my words but sees only one big blur.*
*He talks to me through senses, tells me how he feels,*

*Shares his pain and anger,*
*Tries to break free from all the seals, which tie him down.*
*He wants to know I see him, confused, he can't see me,*
*He needs to know I hear him, try and help to set him free.*
*His screams are just loud noises, to all the people by his side,*
*But to him, they're desperate cries in need,*
*No more tears, too many cried.*
*He rocks his body on his own,*
*Moans in the language only he knows.*
*Knows he is alone, in his silent world,*
*That silent boy, desperate to be found.*

# January 2007

I only realise now, what else has changed within me. Like I've developed obsessions I never used to have. And we're on the road; Demi in the pushchair in front of me, the buggie racing before me, because there's a car one hundred yards beyond us, coming this way and if the buggie isn't on the pavement before it shoots past us behind me then something bad will happen and everything will be ruined.

So I'm pushing it, faster than ever, my heart beating so fast and the adrenaline pumping through me and I can't move any faster or everyone will see me panic so I'm concentrating really hard; trying to look normal and yet save my daughters life at the same time.

And then we're there, and we've made it, we're on the pavement, both of us, so this time I'm safe too and the car goes past us, my back turned to what could have been tragic and I can breathe out, let the fear leave my body and hurry along back to the flat, avoiding the roads as best I can.

It happens when I'm in bed as well though, the fear griping at me, forcing me to do what I have to do every night now; put my soft purple dressing gown on top of me, underneath the duvet. Pull the neckline right up to my chin, cover my arms and my hands, pull it down as far as it will reach to my mid calves and then put the duvet on top of us, making sure it covers my ankles because the dressing gown won't reach that far, and if my feet are bare, he'll chop them off.

So now I'm done, and I'm roasting hot, but I can't open the window or he might get in, so we're baking hot in this stuffy little room, all of us sweating, but Dino understands, and he's made sure the baby is cool and the fan is blowing on the other side of the room and I lay there, certain I'm protected if the dressing gown and the duvet can cover me; knowing it is only me he is after.

So now it makes sense, I've developed a form of OCD – Obsessive Compulsive Disorder, but I mustn't tell anyone about that either or they'll think I'm even crazier.

So I'm using the green high lighter that my brain is telling me I must use. Not the blue one or the pink one that look so pretty on the large paper we're to draw on, just the green one, a green that I've grown to love, or hate. I don't understand it; I just know now everything must be green.

The walls in our bedroom are green, the baby girl I should be dressing in pink needs to wear pale green clothes, and I have to paint my toe nails green, hide them under my socks but knowing that green can protect me, like it's a colour he can't cope with and having green around me will force him away.

And I smile at how ridiculous I sound. Knowing I can't explain this to anyone. Having a fixation with a colour; it's insane and I know it, I just can't deal with it; I just can't change it.

Routine; my routine; I'm suddenly obsessed with it too. Like nothing else is as important as it is and if any of it changes my world is crashing down around me.

Everything has to be the same every day; I need to get out of bed at exactly 7:05 am, so if the baby wakes up at 5:45 we are stuck sitting there for over an hour. Her lying beside me or on my lap, me just waiting for the clock to turn, watching the minutes pass, waiting for my safe time, the time I am allowed to rise.

And it continues throughout the day; that I need to be at my parent's house and if I don't touch base there or miss a day out then I'm in danger again and something bad will happen.

And my eating gets worse, so that now I am allowed to eat, like something inside me told me it would be ok, but still not in front of people, still in secret, so that in the middle of the night I put her back down and in the privacy of our room while Dino sleeps beside us, I scoff my face and hide myself away, feeding my body and the evil inside it.

And it transfers through me to the baby, so that she has to have her bottle at a certain time every few hours and needs to be in bed at exactly seven pm every night and if someone is round I have to practically force them out through the door, or if we aren't in the flat, I need to race back there; 'cause if she misses it, if she's late, everything is ruined and the night will be tragic.

It drives me insane, that every time I go to the toilet I need to use precisely six sheets of toilet paper and fold them a particular way and that whenever I drink I need to take five gulps of liquid before I can stop and I have to vary the amounts of fluid entering my lips so that I have five exact mouthfuls.

But no-one understands these silly little rituals that mean so much to me; so instead, I hide these thoughts as well, pretending on the outside that everything's ok, when really inside my mind feels suffocated and sour.

*****

*You've been gone so long, I'm trying to be strong,*
*But it's difficult without you here beside me.*
*They say time heals, but I'm still here crying,*
*Waiting for your return, still trying to bring you back.*
*I still feel the cold, the bitter wind slapping my face as we ran,*
*Tripping in the snow, not knowing where to go.*
*I'm trying to forget it, they say I can.*
*My hands were numb, we hid and you would hum,*
*Trying to save my mind from the insanity and the fear.*
*"It's so late now, I'll just rest my eyes…" You whisper in the black of the night,*
*"Please don't leave me…." I whisper back,*
*But by the time I awake, it's too late.*
*The shot makes me jump,*
*No doubt about it, I felt the lump, in my throat swell harder,*
*I turn to look at you, I can't move,*
*You're lying there dying, what are they trying to prove?*
*I look for them in the dim light,*
*But I can't see anyone, no-one's in sight.*
*I know I'm crying, but I can't feel anything,*
*I know you're dying, but I can't do anything,*
*I know you've let me here and I'm alone.*
*They say time heals; but that was years ago.*

What's happening to me? Why am I confused about the life I am living? I feel like I'm living different lives. I've

99

got different pasts and different memories I never knew before. I don't know if they're real or not. I don't know the life I used to lead.

# May 2007

I thought I was better when I went back to work, I guess I always knew it was temporary, but I wasn't ready for the day I lost my boy.
Everything came crashing down again; only worse.

I lost Cody in December '06. He went to his special school and although I started work there, I couldn't help him and it just broke my heart to see how downhill he had gone. I don't think I could take much more and before I knew it, I had left.
I told him I was going, I told him I'd never forget him, but whether or not any of it sank in, I really don't know. I couldn't bear to be there, and not work with him, and see him struggling so much.

There were other boys I could have worked with; well, that I tried working with. I think it worked for a while, but then my heart just ran out of the love and kindness I'd always had for them, and my connection with them started to suffer.
I knew I was ill again.

*****

My relationship with Demi had eventually started to

develop. Our bond grew when I had gone back to work, and I started to look forward to seeing her. I bathed her every day and sang and rocked her to sleep. I began to love her more than I ever thought I would. I missed her when I went to work and enjoyed coming home to her, hearing all about what she had done with my Dad during the day.

When I started to suffer again though, so did our relationship. It got to the point where I couldn't stand to be in the new flat.
I thought we'd be happy there, and for a while we were. Demi had her own bedroom and I decorated it with beautiful fairies and princess stickers. But when I got ill, I ended up leaving her in there.
If she cried when teething, I would just shut the door and leave her to suffer the pain alone. I hate remembering that now.
When I'm in pain, I need cuddles, and now I realise that's all she needed, but at the time, my mind couldn't see it like that.
Everything seemed different; so much worse.

So she'd get used to her own company. She had to struggle on through things by herself.
My care for her improved, hence the daily bathing, I changed her nappies more frequently, and didn't avoid doing them as much as I had used to. I cut her nails and started putting her fine hair up in little ponytails.

Her cyst was shrinking and was getting less and less noticeable by the month. I adored to show her off in beautiful thin clothes now, rather than hiding her under layers and layers of warm woolly cardigans and jumpers. She started to crawl and would scuttle across the room to follow me. If I left, she'd cry for hours, or so Dino told me. It was a wonderful feeling, knowing that despite everything we'd been through together, she still loved me.

*****

I weaned her far too late and failed miserably in doing so though. She didn't want anything, bar her bottle. I think at night, when I should have been there cuddling her, she had only her milk bottle to console her and she became ridiculously attached to it.

If I tried to change the milk to water she would scream and hide and refuse to drink to the point where I was terrified she would dehydrate, and if I tried to give her milk in a different bottle or a new cup, the same would happen. She wouldn't sleep without it; she wouldn't be, without it.

So she grew to believe her milk was her mummy, I guess. When I tried to wean her onto yoghurts or mushed up fruit she refused it. She didn't want it and that was that. I began to see a side of Demi that reminded me of myself; her stubbornness.

I tried for months to get her to eat. It would end up in a huge argument with her crying and me forcing spoonfuls of food into her mouth when she blatantly didn't want it. I got worked up and upset. We'd both end up in tears and more often than not I'd end up shouting and screaming at her. Sometimes I told her off, or just went off on one, hurting myself and telling myself what an awful parent I was.

Most of this happened when we were on our own. When my family saw it happening one day, I think they were mortified. Jo had weaned Ady months ago and he had taken so well to it. They all tried to help me, offering to do the feed for me, which generally worked to a degree, but as soon as I tried, as soon as I said the word dinner or picked up the spoon, Demi would clamp her mouth shut or scream and shout.

Sometimes Dino would come home and find us both hysterical. Orange jars of dinner would be slung all over the floor, where she had desperately tried batting them away from her. Her face would be covered and more often than not, she would wretch and vomit most of it back up.

I knew I had failed. I knew I had been too ill to do it properly and this black cloud hung over us both at meal times. I would stuff myself during the day, putting tons of weight on. Making myself feel even uglier and worse than I had before. She wouldn't eat, and we'd go round in circles, making meal times unbearable for us both.

I often took her for dinners at Jos next door. She would sit with Jo and Ady and eat small mouthfuls of whatever Jo prepared. That made me feel even more depressed. No matter what I made for her, she wouldn't eat it. I despised food. I despised meal times, family dinners, even watching her eat other people's food.

I would watch her put each spoonful of Jo's dinner into her little mouth; and I'd wretch inside. I wanted to scream.

She's chewing it and swallowing it and all I want to do is force it all into my own mouth.

I'm gagging on my own meal and I can't eat beside her anymore.

I know if I look at her she'll stop. Part of me wants to stare and force her to stop. Another part of me wants to leave the building so I'm no where near her and she can enjoy her food for a change. That's the part of me that happens. I knew I had to do something to get out of this awful cycle, but I just didn't know what.

*****

"Just eat it! Just eat the food. Let me put the spoon in and just swallow it Demi!" I'm shouting as if it's going to work.

She just starts crying so now I shout "FINE, die of starvation!"

She's eighteen months now and I'm still ill; she still won't eat.

I put my face right up to hers and say "Please, just eat it; now!"

She starts gagging and choking on the spoonful I just forced in her mouth and then she starts to vomit what little food I'd managed to get into her.

As soon as I see it and smell it, I'm heaving myself and have to run to the toilet.

I never used to have this sick phobia. Now it's taking over

my stomach.

So then I'm vomiting myself, and I can hear her crying, so I wipe my mouth and go back to find her covered in her own sick, her face bright red, her eyes stained with tears and looking empty and afraid, and now I feel it again, the guilt, the horridness of what I've done.

So I clean her up, trying not to heave again.

I talk nicely to her.

"Mummy's sorry. I'm sorry darling. I just want you to eat or you'll get poorly" and she's muttering yes and nodding and just reaching out for me to hold her, so I do, and she's naked and breathing heavily and sniffling and then Dino walks in the door and sees us and takes her from me, so I clean up the mess I've just created and Dino gives her the milk and now she's quiet and snuggling up to him and I feel the same stabbing feeling inside.

He comes to me now she's happy and I just shake my head. I'm doing it all wrong, I know I am. He must know too.

She refuses every meal for a reason. I'm the reason. And that makes me hate her eating even more.

"If she won't eat with me, she won't eat at all." I say and leave the room.

It took me two and a half years to get her to eat with me.

*****

The phobia of cooking hasn't disappeared yet. I can't eat indoors, I can't eat food I've cooked or even looked at for too long.

We eat out nearly every day. Our bills are late being paid, we've got red mail, but I can't think about it. I need to get out.

I couldn't cook when I was pregnant, couldn't even stand to look at food in our house, but it didn't go like I thought it would; it got worse.
I had to eat the same meal every single day, part of the OCD maybe; another uncontrollable obsession.

I ate chicken tikka masala four nights a week for four months, and then it had to be pizza, every single day without fail. I piled the weight back on and my health deteriorated even more.

I lived off energy drinks; red bull and coke.
I had to get through the days of being alone, my mind fuzzed up and when I had three or four red bulls; my mind didn't work the same. I was on high mode; constantly moving. I didn't have to lie down and play dead then.

*****

And Demi's older now, yet still sharing her baths with me. A time I feel close to her and not afraid by the nakedness of our bodies like at other times I am forced to fear.
And she's laying in front of me, kicking her legs and throwing her hands up and down on the water, splashing and giggling when the bubbles cover our faces and now I'm smiling because it's so much fun, knowing Dino is only in the other room; here to protect us, just in case, seeing that the curtains are drawn and that this moment is just for us, and any of the unbearable thoughts that

often creep in to my mind are gone, blocked by the water and the privacy of this time.

\*\*\*\*\*

*Daddy,*
*My eyes fill with tears, as I listen to your words,*
*Memories of all our years, chirping like the birds, you*
*listened to before.*
*We listen to his songs, both knowing he is right,*
*Makes me wonder, what my life will be like, when one day*
*you're not around.*
*I look into your eyes Daddy, knowing you are mine,*
*Knowing the time you leave, will be the time, I'll treasure*
*our memories most.*
*Your eyes tell me everything Daddy, they open up your soul,*
*I love to read your thoughts that way,*
*Know they've stayed the same, through youth and old.*
*I look at you now, every day,*
*Watch the way you talk and act,*
*Listen to the things you think and say,*
*Treasuring each word like the gold it's worth.*
*I wish I could thank you for such a wonderful Mum,*
*Now I know how you just always knew, she was the one.*
*I wish I knew how to show you,*
*That without the sister I have,*
*I'd be lost, my family, the life you gave me.*
*I know that your smell, will always be with me,*
*The image of your smile, something I'll never not be able to*
*see,*
*Stuck in my mind, like a vision of a king with his queen.*
*The days are going by now and we're so much older now,*
*I'm sitting here today, trying to imagine how,*

*I'll be ok when you are gone.*
*I'm a younger version of you Daddy and that makes me so*
*proud,*
*That's why we fight and shout, and why I scream out loud.*
*But even when that happens, I know things are still fine,*
*Because you'll always be my Daddy,*
*You're there for me all of the time and I love you for that.*
*Don't think I never think of you,*
*Because I do every day,*
*I remember every minute we've shared,*
*I remember you in every way.*
*I never want to forget those things Daddy,*
*Because they're part of what makes me who I am.*
*I just wanted to say thank you, for being who you are too.*
*Watching over me, to keep me safe,*
*Like the protective shining star that watches Mum.*
*I know sometimes you think I do not care,*
*But I know I'll think of you even when you aren't here.*
*Thank you for singing to me and stroking my hair,*
*And giving me the precious memories, we both now share.*
*I love you more than life itself Daddy and I always will.*

My Daddy's everything right now; he always will be.

# September 2007

So I'd quit my job and stayed at home with Demi. Before I knew it, I was pregnant again. We'd talked about trying again when I'd gotten better, but I don't think either of us realised it would happen so quickly.

I was ecstatic. I was carrying my husbands' baby. Again. This time a boy. We were both elated.
I had very little energy but the depression seemed to lift. I was back on that cloud. The same happy cloud I used to float on when Demi was inside me.

Demi had stopped napping when she was about fifteen months old. I tried to stay awake all day until Dino got home and then I was in bed and asleep by 7pm.
He let me sleep whenever I wanted, for as long as I needed. He watched Demi the whole time, played games with her, fed her, put her to bed...
Their relationship grew so strong. Besides me, they were our unit. Together, they looked after me; they understood me.

*****

And now I find myself thinking of her; my older sister, writing to her, to try and curb her pain; make up for how she hurt all those years ago:

'I wanted to write you this letter because I've been thinking so much about you lately. When you talk to me about Dad leaving it makes me cry inside. It makes me wish I could have helped you or looked after you, or just been there to cuddle you. Sometimes I find it hard to talk about it because I feel guilty and sad because I know Dad hurt you; all of you.

I can't give you any answers because I don't know half of what happened. I can't hate him because he has never hurt me. Part of me understands how much you must hurt inside, if it was us he had left, I would probably feel the same way. Jo said herself that if he went off with a new family, she would never even speak to them.

I know he loves you. So much more than you think he does. He never brushed you away under a carpet like you think he did. He talked about you all the time, the older I've grown, the more he has confided in me. I can't help how close I am to him. I never knew it was different to a relationship you two have.

He told me things about when you were tiny. Talked to me about the day you were born and how poorly you were with anemia. He showed me pictures he has of you and the boys when you were all little and talked about how beautiful you are.
I think he is afraid to talk to you because inside he knows how much he hurt you. He knows you'll never forget what happened and that he hurt his little girl like he

never should have.

I don't know if you remember, but one day when we lived in Stalbridge when I was about 10, I had a row with him and said I was going to run away. I packed a little bag like a stupid little girl and you came upstairs and spoke to me and you told me how silly I was being and how I should be grateful I had a dad there with me. I have very few memories of my childhood, but that is one I will never forget. That day I saw things as they were.

When we moved out I didn't see him very much. Jo lives 20 minutes away but unless they come here, they don't see him either. He doesn't make much effort with anyone. It isn't just you. It isn't that he is different with Jo and me and then you three. If anything at all; it is me segregated from the four of you, and that isn't him favouring me or loving me more.

I have always clung to him, I don't know if it is because I realised what you had lost and I never wanted to lose that or what, but I have never left his side. I moved out, tried to be adult and live with my own separate family but I couldn't do it. I had to come back, just for Dad. I don't love anyone else in the world the way I love him. I love him more than I even ever thought was possible. I would die tomorrow for him. In my eyes, nothing he can do is wrong, nothing, except for one thing. The fact that he left and hurt all of you.

I know that if he gets terribly ill in old age, it will be me washing and bathing him, it will be me wiping his bum if he goes to the loo, I will be his carer just like I am now. My Mum works hard for money for us all, and I know she loves him, but in truth, I think I love him more than anyone else in the world will ever love him; even her.

I am so very sorry that he hurt you, I really truly am. I feel like your sister I really do; I am your sister. I am Jo's sister and I look after her when she is sad. I wish I could have done that for you. I know you lay in bed and cried, I know you did and so does he and I wish to God it never happened. I wish I could have laid with you and held you so you didn't have to be alone, but I can't change it and it kills me inside.

I have a very unique relationship with him. I never realised it was different until Jo and I were in our late teens. I never noticed I was any closer to him than you were, or than Jo is. I only realised a few years ago and it makes me feel terribly guilty. I know he loves me, but I wish you could see how much he loves you too. Sometimes Jo feels the same way you do but she never lets it upset her; that's just the way she is.

Dad is my soul mate; as weird as that might sound. He knows everything about me; all my secrets; and I know his. It's not a normal relationship, I spoke to a psychiatrist about it once and they were really concerned.

I could write his autobiography for him I know him that well. I love every hair on his head and I will never ever see any bad in him. It tears me up knowing though, that he is capable of hurting people the way he hurt you. Please understand that he loves you so much. You were his first little girl; his princess - his saucepot.

He is getting old now and really ill and he lives every day with what he did to you. He never wants you to stop loving him and he will never stop loving you. I don't think he believes he will be here for many more Christmases and he wants this one to be about coming to see all of you. There's no other reason why he would be so adamant about me not coming. I offered to pay for our own train fairs and accommodation but he said it's not about that. He wants to see you. If you don't talk to him you'll never know how he feels. I don't know if it matters to you anymore; I just wish there was something I could do. I love you so much. I know we aren't as close as we could be; I wish we were. XXXXX'

And my eyes are streaming, with the knowledge of what happened, the sadness I feel inside for her, because she was his poppet, she was his princess, and she still is, but she doesn't realise it.

*****

*Dark roads ahead, that I'm too afraid to walk down, alone now, my hand is cold.*
*My head is full of thoughts, so loud,*
*But outside, life is so silent, so cold, I'm numb.*
*My fingers pale, my lips blue, cheeks, skin, like ice,*
*Feel so deep down, below Earth, all alone, trapped.*
*Afraid to breathe, can't breathe, no need.*
*I see myself, separated, my soul stares at my body, icy tears trickle and freeze.*
*My body has no feeling.*
*But suddenly, heat burns through my hand,*
*Your fingers enclose mine, you smile and share your*

*warmth,*
*Body recovers heat, blood flow,*
*Normal colour, ice melts.*
*I am part of you; kiss my lips, no longer blue.*

# February 2008

I'm not ready for this. I'm sitting in my Granny's house. Demi's asleep in the travel cot. My darling Granny just died.

I phoned Dino and tried not to cry as I told him what had happened. He told me to stay calm because it wasn't a good idea to get stressed or distraught when I was seven months pregnant.

I hung up the phone and cuddled my Mum. She was devastated. It was written all over her face. We were shocked. I felt like I was in a dream; and I start to wonder, how do you explain something like this to a child?

I went into the bedroom and stroked her beautiful golden hair. She was snoring as usual and I just let the tears flow down my face.

"It's always you poppet, isn't it? It's always you who is here for me...."

I whispered to her that GG is a star now; same as her baby brother and sisters.

I stroked my huge bump and collapsed onto the bed. I didn't know how I'd ever fall asleep.

I must have though, because the next thing I know, I'm being woken by the strangest noise, like there's a train going right past the house? I'm sure I'm shaking. No, the house is shaking. The whole house is moving and vibrating.

What the hell is happening??? Granny?? Dad?? I'm trying to call out but no-one can hear me.

I leap out of bed and run into the other room. I stand frozen in the doorway, unable to move any further. All the furniture in the bedroom is moving. I'm so confused.

Then just as quickly as it starts; it stops.

I go straight to my Dad's side and shake him awake. I tell him to sit up as I need to talk to him about something very serious.

He tries to wake himself up and turns the light on while sitting himself beside me.

Mum is still fast asleep.

I try and explain what just happened but he won't believe me. I think he thinks' I've finally gone round the bend.

"I am telling you Dad, the house was literally moving..."

He grips my hand and sighs deeply.

I think I end up going back to bed, almost convinced I imagined it. Surely I didn't dream something like that, did I??


And then I wake up again, and its morning and it seems more real than ever. And it says on the tele, first earthquake in twenty-five years and my jaw drops because I didn't imagine it and I wasn't dreaming and Dad is just staring at me in shock.

And all I can think about is thank God I am alive. Thank God my baby is ok and Demi was right here beside me like she always is.


And I no longer feel scared about my Granny. I think she

wanted to tell us something, and she sure as hell did with an Earthquake a matter of hours after she died.

Suddenly I'm not afraid, and the feeling of worry just fades. I know things will be ok once I've had the baby. She will look after me and so will everyone else.

Something invisible confirms it.

*****

I look around the rooms, busy with belongings that they've always had, and yet now they feel empty.

I can still smell my Granny on everything; her clothes I hold to my face, the towels, even the sofa.

Suddenly everything is precious.

I have to handle everything with extra care, like if I break it now, she'd be devastated.

I place the ring she left me on my right hand.

Three beautiful diamonds, perfectly complimenting the engagement ring on my other hand.

I twist it and turn it and smile at how it fits my finger perfectly; and I thank her, thank her for leaving me such a beautiful sentiment of our relationship.

I glance at my Grandfathers certificates on the wall; finger his war medals lovingly.

I've never looked at his possessions before. I wish I had because now they are tarnished with the knowledge of what he did.

*****

We decide to move back in with my parents. Just in case

the Post-Natal Depression comes back. I want to go home more than anything. I've never been ready to leave.

It feels like a huge weight has been lifted.

We're all together like we should be.

I wish Jo and Skip could be here. My family need to all be together.

I got so close to her in the flat; she was my baby sister, my best friend, and my next door neighbour. Now she feels like an acquaintance; a stranger.

I can't think about that now though; I have to push the feeling of missing her away.

I need to think about Demi, and the baby, and Dino and me.

I need to be where I am safe, and happy.

I need to protect us from what nearly destroyed us all before.

It feels right the day we move in.

Dino is sad to leave the flat he loves so much, and part of me feels guilty because I know I'm tearing him away from that, but at the same time I know he'll be happy if me and the kids are.

And we really are.

Demi had always called my Dad, Dad.

Dino's not too keen on that, but I love it.

I want my kids to love him as much as I do.

He's always protected me; always looked after me and loved me and never ever let anyone hurt me.

I want him there for my kids; always.

That's why I know she's safe when she's with him.

*****

Mum and I are driving; driving to the sea front so I can feel safe again.

The water is so calm; I can just see it softly swaying, back and forth, in the dim lit light of the moon and the houses shining down on it.

I'd told Mum I needed a walk, she'd practically laughed at me.

"You're not going anywhere; not this late, not on your own!" And she's staring at me, speaking to me like a tiny little girl, like the one I sometimes feel haunts me.

"I'm not a child Mum. I wasn't asking for your permission; I was making a statement." And my jumpers on and I'm almost out the door, when she tells me she'll drive me and we can go to the sea together.

She tells me how afraid she is, to let me be alone, she tells me that I'm ill and that I can't have the opportunity to hurt myself anymore. That they let us move back in, so that they could protect me and look after me, on the days that destroy me like right now.

And then we are there, sitting in silence, for probably the twenty-third time this month, because it's become another obsession, that I have to come here, I need to; or I might die inside if I don't touch base with 'home-ground'.

When we drive back, I see a woman, rush along the road in front of us; she hurries because we're approaching, though Mum isn't going fast at all. Obviously she passes the car, but I watch her, and I see that we have passed her before she has reached the pavement.

'You're dead.' I think inside....certain that because she never made it to the curb the devil is going to get her.

And then I'm deeply concerned; thinking only of her, and reminding myself of the importance of my 'obsessions' for the remainder of the journey home.

# April 2008

It's hurting so much - I haven't even gotten a chance to realise I'm in labour before contractions are rippling through my lower abdomen; crippling me if I try and stand up.

No-one believes me when I say I'm in agony. I guess they all think it will be like it was with Demi.

Finally I've got some gas and air, and then the world seems to change in a matter of seconds.

It doesn't feel like pain anymore; not to the same degree.

My head is spinning and my whole body feels heavy and yet numb at the same time.

At first I feel sick and emotional but then it starts to hit me and my throat is dry already.

And then Jo is there; staring right at me; talking me through the pain while the woman internally examines me; bringing back jet black nightmares; making me rigid with terror; breathless with the fear and the memories.

I'd never remembered before; I'd never known what had happened; why I was so sad, why I was so uncomfortable with myself down there.

But now I knew; because when her fingers were pressing the tip of my cervix, I felt a stab in my heart; like she had pushed her hand right up through me to my chest and was trying to rip it out the other end.

Suddenly, the world seemed to slow down. Everything was silent except I could actually hear my own heart beating.
I was listening to a boom boom, boom boom, without realising it was me.

And Jo's eyes are watery; they're shining in the light. She's holding my hand and I think that just by staring in her eyes, she can see into my soul like no-one ever has.
Because there she is again, prodding at my insides, reminding me of how I was robbed of this privacy before; bringing nasty memories flooding back; confusing me at the very worst time.

Jo though, Jo is there. The only person I could possibly have wanted, to so unknowingly, share this tender moment with me.

And then her fingers are out; and I realise I'd stopped breathing in the gas, and the room is loud and busy again and I can hear everything normally, only now it feels too much; too loud for my ears and I know I'm grimacing; I'm writhing in agony, yet I feel so deadly still, and I don't want to take my eyes off Jo; I don't want this moment to end, because never before have I felt so close to her....

*****

My pregnancy with the baby had gone well. We didn't have any major concerns like Demi's cyst or the way he was lying and the labour was completely different.

My waters broke and the following day I had Scott-Connor, completely naturally without an epidural or any blood transfusions. I needed stitches again, but I recovered so quickly.

Dino and Mum said to me the evening he was born, "God, you don't look like you've just had a baby at all, you look fantastic!"
Truth was; I felt fantastic!
I had a boy. I'd always wanted a boy.

He was gorgeous, everything I could have hoped for. And as much as I loved Demi being the spit of Dino, it was nice to a have a baby that resembled me, if even only slightly.
He was perfect; absolutely perfect.

*****

Something changed inside me the day he was born.
I missed her. I missed Demi so much more than I thought I would. I missed washing her hair and spending time drying it and brushing it. I missed helping her do colouring, or playing building blocks with her. I wanted to go home; to her.
Dino would visit every day, I could see that he adored Scott; it was obvious to everyone. He had a son now; he was overjoyed.

Demi though. My Demi.
I spoke to her on the phone, all the time. I thought about her, every second I was away from her.
And suddenly it dawned on me what had happened;

what I had done to her; what I had put her through, throughout the last two years of my depression.

And then she was there. Running up the hallway towards me. Skipping and looking back over her shoulder, calling to Dino to hurry up, 'cause there was Mummy. And she was shouting me. Running past all the other women, the new mummies or the midwives. And I was so proud. This was my baby. MY little girl. I couldn't stop smiling. She was back; and to think I really could have lost her.
"Mummy!!!" She screeched, running into my arms. I scooped her up and was gobsmacked at the size of her. She was huge; she looked massive compared to this tiny little bundle....my son.
"I missed you so much Demi" I whispered, and before I knew it, I found myself choking back the tears.

Dino sorted the baby into his car seat, as today we got to go home, but all I wanted to do, all I needed, was my baby girl.
Because somehow, something had changed. I'd fallen more in love with her than I could have ever imagined.
I could see it all now. I could see what had happened. I could picture it from both sides. Mine; where my mind seemed to die, and then my darling daughters' side, who had suffered every moment alongside me.

*****

And then I find myself thinking of my Granny. Wishing she could have met my son; sad that she could have held on for just a few more weeks to meet him and hold him like she held my daughter and held me all those years ago. And I wish she was back, sitting beside me on the orange sofa in her lounge, watching millionaire on the tele, stroking my hands in hers.

So I twiddle the ring she gave me around my finger, holding it in the light so the diamonds shine up at me, and I'm smiling, 'cause I know she's with me, has been every day since her body left this world; her soul watching over me; over him, forever.

# November 2008

I'm so lucky. He's the most wonderful baby.
He smiles all day long; never cries.
He sleeps and he gurgles.
He loves me and he cuddles me and makes me happy.
I can enjoy being with him.
I don't have to sit up all night with him. When he falls back to sleep, so do I.
I don't have the nightmares anymore.
For a while it feels like it's gone.
I'm on the tablets again anyway.
I still feel sad but I don't ever think about hurting him.
It's still all me and Demi.

It hurts so much inside; surely this will make it all stop now.
I'm walking in the rain and the dark.
Demi's sitting on top of Scotty in the buggie. Her legs are wrapped round him and he's fallen asleep.
I'm freezing and soaked through.
They both look like little Snowmen; wrapped up in their coats, blankets, hats, gloves and scarves.
They're so quiet and calm.

Demi isn't even asking me what's going on; she probably already knows.

My phone's flashing in the dark; it makes me remember the day my Dad was ringing me before.

You can't save me today Daddy; I'm not going to let you.

I shove it in my pocket on silent and forget about the people at home.

I wanted to leave a note; I wanted to let everyone know I loved them, but I couldn't, that would force me to think about them.

People are all around me, I didn't think the streets would be this busy.

Suddenly I feel like everyone is watching me; staring at me. They must all know where I am going.

I need to change direction.

We're going to the ocean I tell Demi.

She loves the ocean.

She came with Dad and I every day to look at the white horses and the choppy waves.

Dad would be thinking about his Grandma and I would be thinking about my babies and we'd both just sit there and share a silent grief that no-one else could understand.

So now I have to go back.

It's the only way I can be with my babies; all of them.

I know Dino's at home; crying.

I know he's run out of things to say and do.

It's making me angry that he doesn't care. He's not ringing me; but my daddy is.

And then it hits me; dad is probably sitting there crying

too.

I know how his mind works; he will be worried sick and then it makes me cry too; for doing this to him, for putting them all through it again.

That's why it has to end this time. No-one will have to worry anymore. No-one will have me as this awful burden pressing down on them every single day.

I can't leave my kids though; Dino told me that would be selfish and that I'd never do it; so I have to take them with me; they need to come and be with my other babies; they need to lie with their siblings they never got to meet; all together with me; in

my arms; in the depths of the ocean; swimming freely; without a single care in the world.

And suddenly I'm sitting; I'm on a bench, crying, and I've pulled Demi into my arms and I'm rocking us both, holding her in to me, telling her everything's going to be ok now.

Then I see my friend's brother. What a funny happening.

I dry my tears and he makes some chit-chat, and it's so odd how I can pretend everything is ok and he doesn't have a clue what's going on in my head; because now I'm able to hide it; all the years of perfecting hiding my pain and my thoughts and then he's gone, and suddenly I'm confused, and I hate myself even more, because I don't know who I am anymore. I don't even know who I am.

But then the car is there; I can see it coming and I need

to move.

I'm jay walking; if I run they'll spot me.

Not that they can miss me; huge and bulging; pushing a ridiculous bundle of kids and crap that I shoved in the bags around it, and I know they can see me.

I have to keep walking though, and then the cars stopped; it's right ahead of me.

And I'm going to walk past it because I can't bear to look at my Daddy right now.

But it's Mum.

It's my Mum who jumps out and runs to me.

And she's shouting, and I think she's going to hit me, but she just runs to me and throws her arms around me and holds me like she's never going to let me go and then I'm sobbing, and she doesn't even have to say anything, neither of us do, because we both know, we both understand and nothing needs to be said.

"Get in the car; get these babies in the car!' And she's pulling at me, dragging us to the car.

I know people are watching us, but I don't care. I don't even care that they probably all know what's happening, because no matter how much I try and hide what is happening to me, it's like my mind is screaming to everybody around.

I'm trying to resist, I just want to go the ocean Mum.

And she knows; she knows why.

She tells me she'll take me there, so we get in the car.

The kids are in the back, and they're warm now.

And Mum just sits at the steering wheel crying. And I have to turn away, because if I look at anybody else's tears, the guilt rips my insides up and it makes me want to die even more.

She's on the phone now, to Dad.

I can't go home Mum, I just can't do it anymore.

So she's driving me. We're going to the ocean. And she hands me a cigarette because she knows they calm me down.

And I'm puffing on it, breathing in the toxins that I know are poisoning my body even more.

I'm not cold now, it's hot in the car, and she's got the heat blowing so the kids can warm up.

And I think Demi's fallen asleep in the back, it's past her bedtime and she's probably exhausted.

And then we're there; and I can see the water; I can hear the waves crashing, like they're angry I never made it to them.

All I can think is that my babies are in there; right there when we put the roses for them, the roses that symbolise their being, and that I should be in there with them.

"Your babies are in the car Rachel; your babies are here with you..." Mum knows what I'm thinking, like she can read through every silent tear that falls.

And I can't even turn to look at them, 'cause I know she is right, and my head is in my hands 'cause I'm so ashamed, so embarrassed and humiliated and now I need to go home; I need to put them to bed, where they should be. Dino is so angry, but he never shows it.

He's been out to every train station. I told him we were leaving. But he didn't know I meant to the ocean; not like my Daddy knew.

And then I'm guilt stricken even more. Because he does care; and just because he didn't phone me the way my Dad does, he went out, he searched for me and his babies; his family that I so nearly stole from him.
I can't be with him. I can't let him hold me in his arms again.
It feels like we're going round in circles. He must be so sick of it.

I'm trying to explain I just wanted to stop his pain, stop destroying his life the way this evil is destroying mine, but he's not listening, he tells me that going away from him, taking the babies we were lucky enough to have, that would destroy him.

And I know he's right, I know I need to change, I know I need to get rid of all this black that's seeping through me, but I don't know how.
I'm trying to tell him, it's like a thick fog that my mind just can't escape from, and he tells me I need to go back to the doctors, I need to tell them how I'm feeling and I'm shaking my head because the thought of telling someone how my mind is just terrifies me, but I know he's right, and I know it has to be done.

I need to lie down; my body feels weak. I'm shaking now, but I don't feel cold.
I just need to curl myself up.

And then I find myself thinking of God.

A God I've never met, never let into my life before, never even debated existing and it's like he's talking to me, trying to heal my pain and I just cry to him, I just ask him to help me, because I've run out of other options, I've run of asking for help from people that just don't know how to.

*****

I'm sitting in the lounge, my Daddy's asleep in his chair. Demi is beside him, leaning on his warm body. Scotty is on my lap; smiling up at me, like he always does and the anger I often feel subsides. I'm not cross that he's smiling anymore.

I kiss his cheeks and stick my tongue out and wish I could have done this for Demi.

She huddles closer to the man who did though, the Daddy bear that looked after her when I couldn't, but I'm not bitter now, because if there had to be someone, anyone that could have protected her when it was needed most, I would choose him, a thousand times over.

The nursery rhymes are playing on the tele, she's engrossed in them, her mind working over-time like it always has done and she's rocking her body along to the music, glancing over at me; checking I'm ok, like she always has done.

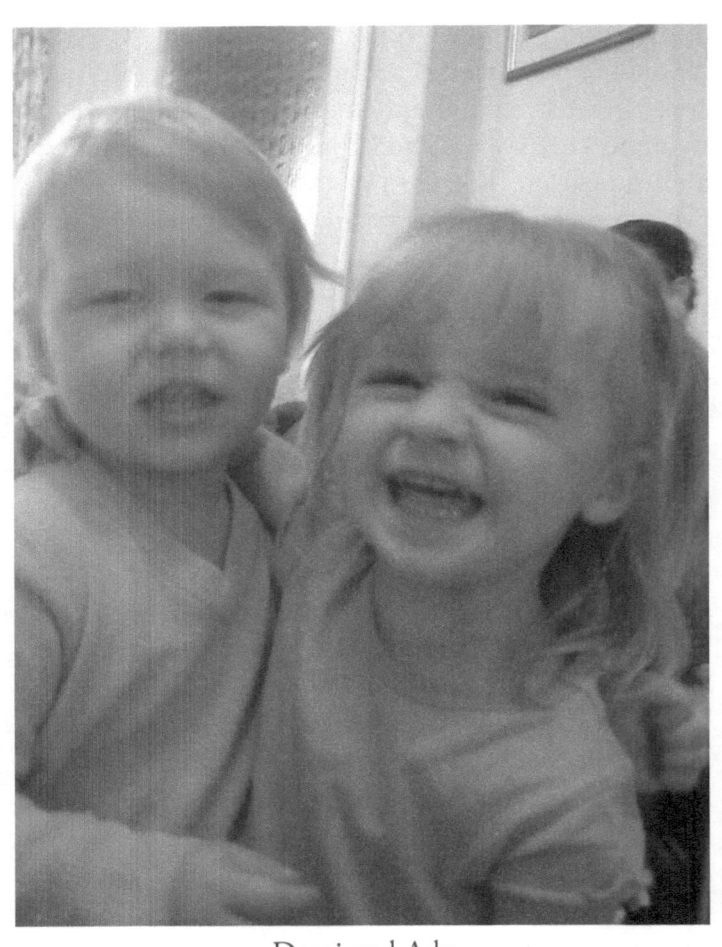

Demi and Ady

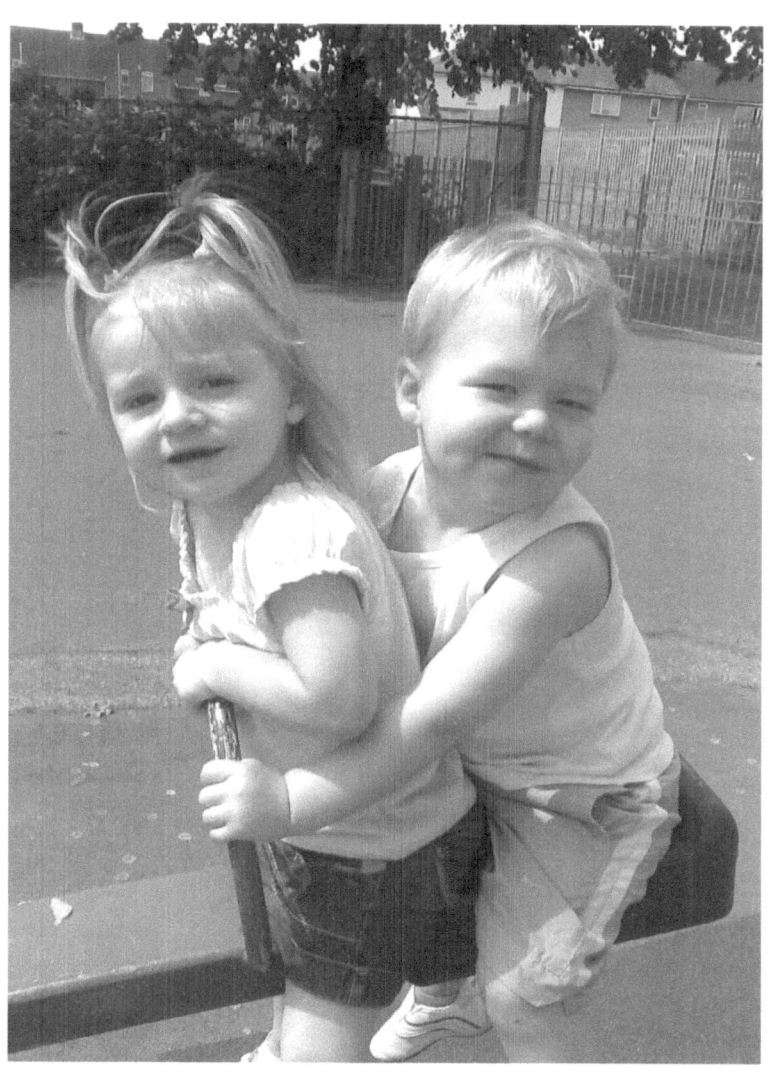

Adrian and Dem

# December 2008

Scotty was growing so fast. I couldn't keep up. He slept all through the night since about four months old and never cried, not even if he was hungry. He was a dream baby. He weaned perfectly at roughly six months, and he took to all sorts of food and piled on the weight.

It was wonderful for my self esteem, I felt so proud. I could succeed. This could work.

He slept in Demi's room as soon as he slept all night and when he did wake, if he was teething, Dino would comfort him. Dino did a lot more for Scott than he did for Demi. I think the post natal depression with her, threw all of us....


I remember waking so many times over those nights, seeing Dino getting up and down; settling and re-settling Scott; comforting him if his gums were hurting; night after night after night.

He never asked me to do it. Not once.

I'd done nearly every night with Demi, and I think deep inside, I was terrified to do them with Scott.

I would sit up for hours after I'd fed her and put her back down. She'd fall straight off to sleep after her milk, but I'd end up just sitting there; thinking.

My mind would start wondering; I'd get horrible flashbacks and nasty thoughts. I was too afraid to sleep incase the nightmares were even worse.

I just lay there; watching them both sleep; my Dino and my Demi. They looked so peaceful and so beautiful.
On many occasions I thought about just walking out the door. Just walking and walking in the dark until eventually I'd lost myself...

*****

I'm sitting on the grass in Wick Lane; watching the ducks floating and the light from the sun reflecting on the shallow water.
Demi's sitting beside me, munching on some crisps, gobbling them up, quiet and satisfied.
She's warm today. She's got her hat and scarf on, wrapped up in a beautiful thick cardie my dads first wife has kindly knitted for her.
Its cold, but we feel good today.

Scotty's on my lap, warm in his new fuzzy coat. Drowning him in length, the hood with little ears covering his head. I'm holding him in to me, shaking the rattle that's resting on his legs and talking to him about the birds and the squirrels; talking to my baby boy like I'd never spoken to Demi.
And he's kicking his legs with excitement and munching on an organic biscuit, because that's what he eats, proper food for my boy.

Demi's smiling at him and jumping up and down now to make him laugh and she's making such a funny face that both of us start to giggle.

This moment feels wonderful. I love this river almost as much as I love the Head. Because Daddy brought me here too; sitting in the car, looking out at the tiny boats along the river bank, watching the blue tits and the finches' fluttering from branch to branch.

*****

It was the first Christmas we'd had as the three of us. We spent it back at home, where we should have been.
It was hard without my Granny, the first Christmas I'd had all my life without her, my sons first Christmas; never having met her.
But it was wonderful. There wasn't a grey cloud hanging over me anymore; now it was going; fading as the weeks went by.

*****

Scotty's always wheezing and coughing and the doctor says he might develop asthma. I hate listening to him breathing like that; like there's something nasty pressing down on his lungs, suffocating him when I can't protect him.
So I give him his inhaler, a big orange tube for such a little guy, but he breaths through it for me, like he knows it is helping and then I feel better, imagining he's getting the feelings I got with gas and air and then his lungs have filled with a good air, a clean air, toxins really, but that help him like I can't.
And then I vow, only to myself, that I'll never light another cigarette again. I know I can do it, because I never smoked with either of their pregnancies, Like I can

switch the desire, the craving for the nicotine that seems to calm my veins, on and off when my brain decides; so now I've decided, no more smoking, not near me, not near my babies. I waver why, and convince myself, some of the evil lies within them, and turning myself away from them, can protect us even more.

# January 2009

I had been thinking for some time about whether to have Demi's IQ tested. The health visitor and psychologist I'd spoken to were both for it, so after talking things through with Dino, we decided we'd go for it.

We all knew she was advanced, but when her IQ came back as 140 and the psychologist said she was gifted, I think my jaw dropped to the ground. GIFTED? Are you insane, I asked him, desperately wanting him to double check all the answers?
He was sure. She was 'very superior' as the tests indicated.
I was shell-shocked; unbelievably proud; jumping up and down with the shock and the amazement that I felt inside.

Demi, at two years old, was recognised as 'gifted'.
I decided things had to change. We needed to do more for her.
I'd spent all of her life so far, making everything about me. Focusing on me, how I felt, what I wanted, what people could do for me.
Now it was time for her. Now after over two years, we needed to make Demi's life, about Demi.

She started various pre-schools and different groups including ballet and music sessions. She loved to read and sing and dance and she played with Scotty every day; we never, ever, had problems with either of them. She was never jealous; she was never mean. I think the worst thing she did was poke him in the eye once, but I think that was more of a test to see what happened rather than to deliberately hurt him!

Sometimes it hurt me that people gave us funny looks and made me feel like it was something I had to hide. A secret like it was something we should have been ashamed of and it used to make me sad; sad that people would think she wasn't 'normal' and annoyed that if she had some sort of special need people would take us seriously, but no-one seemed to care or want to help her like I did. I hoped that would change when she started school.

So for now, I'd just sit with her, reading through the workbooks she'd asked me to buy; helping her do puzzles and talking about the moon; the planets that lived in the sky, the countries on the Earth; all of it fascinating her.

The health visitor helped us; made me feel like my daughter is good and accepted and special like I think she is and then she'd helped us, understood us, making me feel like it was ok that Demi is clever. Not like the pre-school made me feel, like it was something we should hide or ignore. She told me everyone would end up hating Demi if she was a 'clever-clogs' but I never meant it like that. I wasn't bragging, I was just so proud.

I wasn't trying to boast and show her off, I just wanted it to be known by the professionals so they could help her and stimulate her like I need to at home. But they let us down, they let me down and more importantly, they let her down.

So for now, we will sit at home and I'll help her like right now only I can. And if she wants to sit and watch cartoons that's fine, but if she wants to talk to me about the phases of the moon or the difference in country sizes, I'll talk to her about that too

Because I spent too long ignoring her and now I'm going to make up for it; provide her with every opportunity I can; like a good Mother should. And I will be a good Mummy; so she can grow up and know what I did in the first few years of her life, and know what I did after that. Know that I got better and I did it just for her; made my life about her; being good, all of it, just for her.

＊＊＊＊＊

I ran out of pills several times over the months after Scotty was born. I was too afraid to go back and ask for more; too humiliated to speak to the snotty women on the other end of the surgery number.

So I used to go without for a few days. I told myself I was trying to come off them; I'd test my body without them. I wasn't ready though; ever. And I'm still not now.I used to hate to admit that but now I don't mind so much. It's who I am now.

It's been two days since I had them. Doesn't sound much, but it would stiff affect me.. My head is dizzy and I'm so nauseous I'm convinced I'm going to be sick. I keep snapping at people and so far I've had a huge argument with Dino and managed to break my Dad to tears.

It's my turn now though, and I start to cry again. Only

now I'm not alone. I'm sitting in the lounge, sobbing for all to hear. I don't need to hide my sadness anymore, because I'm lucky enough to have a family full of people that understand me now. Dino puts his arms around me without even uttering a word. He apologises for upsetting me, when we both know it's not his fault. It makes me cry harder 'cause I know how desperate he is for me to be the person I used to be'; though I think we are both starting to accept that perhaps I just never will be.

*****

Demi's looking at me from across the room. She tottles over to me, and flings her arms round my neck.

"You crying Mummy? Don't cry!" and she squeezes her cheeks together to try and make me smile. When it only half works, she beeps the end of my nose and starts to sing Twinkle Twinkle, which is the song I sing to her whenever she is hurt or crying.
Inside I want to cry harder; she is so beautiful, and so special. She knows I'm sad, and she's racking her brain for ways to make me happy again; just like her Daddy.

I sit up and dry my tears. There's a lump in my throat where I'm not done crying, but I swallow it and force myself to laugh so she feels better and instantly her look changes and she goes back to playing with her kitchen.

I walk over to her and cup her face in my hands.
"You are so beautiful Demi Day, and so special. You're my princess and don't you EVER forget that!" She smiles up at me and says, "Yeah Mummy. I love you so much!" and

I'm happy now. The sadness has disappeared for another day.

*****

And soon we are running, darting up the pavement to the shop; because she loves to run, like it makes her feel free as a bird. And I ask her to hold my hand, so I can run along side her, but she's smiling and running faster, loving the new feeling of independence she has developed.

"I want to do it myself Mummy. I want to walk on myself like a big girl." And I'm smiling as I chase after her, pretending to catch her, and dragging her up in to the air beside me; smothering her with kisses. And it reminds me of when we're at home, how she insists on brushing her own teeth, washing her own hair, putting herself to bed and wanting to butter her own toast. And I love what a brave girl she is, how she wants to be independent, and I imagine her as a woman, with her own children one day; loving them the way I love her; unconditionally.

And I think, as she is running ahead of me, to the park now, her face covered with a huge smile, how far we have come. How distant we were from this day two years ago and how only now, I can see things clearly. And then it hits me again, like a bolt of lightening through my veins, the sensation of love overpowering me, reminding me of the day I first saw her on the screen at my six week scan, a tiny bean, and the feeling of adoration returns, without warning, like it does most days now; piercing my insides in the most wonderful way.

Then my mind has wandered and I'm thinking of all the children that don't have the privileges she is lucky enough to now have, and I think of how they are all over the world, parentless, starving, cold and alone and I decide that very moment to help with the charities I've been talking with and I know Dino will support me when I tell him how we need to give them twenty percent of our savings and my smile has broadened even more; knowing I can give back to the world that constantly gives to me.

*****

It's her bedtime, seven in the evening; always has been. And she's cosy in her covers, covered in pictures with Spanish writing beside them, because that's the language she loves, and we're looking at the moon on her wall; she's using the buttons to change it's phases and she's loving looking at the light, talking to me about how the crescent changes. And then she's yawning, rubbing her tired eyes, so I lie her down and sing her favourite song to her, stroke her hair back off her face and caress her beautiful soft skin.
'Twinkle, twinkle, little star,
How I wonder what you are.
Up above the world so high,
Like a diamond in the sky.
Twinkle, twinkle, little star,
How I wonder what you are!'
Soon she's asleep but I'm still sitting there, humming the song she adores, wondering if the calm it brings her is drifting in to her dreams too.
And then I'm up, moving slowly from the room; the same room I lay in when I lost my first baby, and I move back to our own room, the room my husband lies in with our son, and I lay beside them, now stroking my babies hair, kissing his cheeks and pulling him in to me.

Dad and I are at Southbourne coast; sitting in the car watching the water swish in and out…hitting the shore like it's teasing the sand and then retreating back again; ever so gently on this lovely calm down.

We can see the Head to our left; murky in the mist; fishermen out on their boats; their orange coats bright in the fog; seagulls flying over them; their white feathers blurring in to the mackerel sky.

There are cars all around us today; they're not usually here. Dad and I talk about how only we are faithful to this place, to the water that belongs to just us.

And the music is pumping from the car stereo and Demi has clambered in to the front on to my lap like she used to, a year ago, and she's pointing out to the sea, to the boats that are floating ever so gently and she listens as Dad talks to me about how good it feels to sit on the sand and feel the pebbles between your toes.

Then we are out; Demi and I, beside the car now, running along the car park; running and laughing and loving the sea air that surrounds us. And Dad is looking at Point house Café; wondering if it's open today like it was all those years ago.

Reminding me that he owned that beach; being the first one there at sunrise and the last one there waiting for the sun to set.

But we're tired from our fun, so we move back off towards the left; turning the car and moving gradually towards our Head.

And then we're there; circling the car park, finding the perfect space, a spot that we can relish in, staring at the beauty of what lies before us. Dad reminiscing to the child he used to be; making dens in all the bushes, rhododendrons either side of him; digging in the sandy earth, finding tiny fossils and stones he could finger lovingly. Telling me of the grass that used to thrive, that's cordoned off now for protection.

We're looking at the fence that surrounds it; the one that wasn't there five decades ago and he's telling me of how he used to climb the sides, scrambling up the rocks to the top where he could look out beyond him and see Christchurch Bay glistening in the distance.

And I'm feeling so good today; thoroughly enjoying listening to him living through the boy he used to be.

*****

I can hear them screaming; both my babies, crying out hysterically from upstairs. I've put the bottles down and I'm racing up the stairs; greeted by Dino at the top cradling Scotty in his arms, his face bright red, and his lips tight with fury.

And Demi is lying on the bed, sobbing, her face covered in tears, her mouth open wide, screaming. Her eyes are shining in the light, staring up at me, glossy, begging me to come to her.

"What happened?" I demand; desperate to know why my babies were so sad.

Demi had jumped backwards on the bed, the back of her skull crashing down onto Scottys forehead.

I turn back to him and see it blue and bruised already. I want to hold him, but Demi is hysterical and Dino is angry, shouting, because he'd just told her not to mess about.

So I've grabbed her. I can't speak. I've just pulled her up

in to me and I'm rushing away, racing down the stairs until we're alone in the lounge.

And I'm holding her now; cradling her in my arms, wrapping my dressing gown around her and singing to her; her favourite song…

She's sniffling and hyperventilating and I'm whispering to her now.

"It's ok baby. Calm down. It's ok, Mummy's here. It was an accident wasn't it. Shhhh…..there there baby…. Mummy's right here…."

And she's stopped crying, she's just nuzzling in to me, burying her head in my bosom and it dawns on me again how much I love her, how protective I am of her, how I can never let her cry, like she used to in her cot when I left her there, unable to think, let alone comfort her.

So we calm down and we go back upstairs, and now Dino holds me, and he soothes me from the stress he knows I feel inside. And he takes Demi from me, drawing her in to him, making her giggle and laugh and checking the back of her head for any lumps.

And I pick up my baby, my brave little man, who's smiling up at me, past it already. And I squeeze him tight and kiss his big blue bruise and apologise for not being up there with them to be there for them when they hurt.

But it's Demi I'm glancing at now, and I need her back on my lap, in my arms where she belongs. And I'm soothing her again, my heart crying inside, for hearing her scream and cry like that tears me up so painfully.

And I know I love her now. Love her more than I ever thought I would.

# Now

I'm listening to Dino's CD, his favourite music; Elton John.
I'm listening to the lyrics of the songs he says are mine.

'I hope you don't mind, I hope you don't mind, that I put down in words, how wonderful life is, while you're in the world...'

And I'm smiling.
My eyes are glossy and I can feel tears pricking them; but good tears; happy tears.
My babies are in my arms.
My mind is wandering to the day I sat in the O2 Arena three months ago with Dino; watching Elton John sing....
holding his hand, feeling so very good inside.

'And all I ever needed was the one
Like freedom fields where wild horses run
When stars collide like you and I
No shadows block the sun
You're all I've ever needed
Baby you're the one'
I don't think my heart has ever felt so swollen with love.
I can't feel it anymore; I can't feel the evil inside me.
I think it's finally gone; it's left me, just as suddenly as the

day it first arrived
.

I am devoting my life to my husband; Dino Day.
The man that loved me right from the start, that never strayed, that never wandered.
The man that loved me for every minute, through every second of pain, every single tear that fell, he kissed away.
We're together again, entwined in the love that first bonded us.
He's my other half; he's the other half of my heart that used to be broken.
My broken heart; he fixed it.

And I'm glancing at my engagement ring; twisting it around my finger; pressing it against the wedding ring that bonds our hearts forever.
Watching the diamond glint in the light, thinking of the words engraved inside the band.
I have never loved him before as much as I do today.

And Scotty's staring up at me. His big beautiful eyes locking with mine and no-else invades this moment. A special time for just us; me and my tiny son and I've not experienced this before; this feeling of love that's over taking me so immediately.

When I look down at him, all I see is my Father. I am so blessed and so happy. My daughter resembles the man I love, my partner for life, like we're swans, free in the stream, forever together. And now I have a son, a baby boy that looks so much like my Daddy and I'm smiling, stroking the thin strands of hair that cover his fragile head and brimming with smiles and a new happiness inside of me.

And then Dino is lying beside me, and we're embracing, I'm drawing him in to my body, trying to join us as one, crushing his body to mine, my heart pounding with love and desire and it feels like I've found a new love that died two years ago, but now it's back and it's stronger than ever and he's whispering how he loves me and missed me and he's smiling because he knows I'm back now, the old me; the Rachel he thought he'd lost forever.

And then he's kissing me, a long kiss that we haven't shared for so many months and his hands are in my hair, on my neck, caressing me and loving me with each touch. And then he's inside me again, filling my body with pleasure and love, and I'm welcoming him into me, my legs parted, not clamped shut like they used to be; forcing him away.
'For each man in his time is Cain
Until he walks along the beach
And sees his future in the water
A long lost heart within his reach'

*****

"You happy Mummy? You happy today?" Demi is staring at me with her gorgeous big grey-green eyes. I'm looking into them, drowning in her soul.
"Yes baby, Mummy's real happy today!" She smiles and flings her arms around my neck.

My relationship with Demi had suffered like no other.

151

We grew to love each other. There was no initial bond, on either part.

We argued, we screamed at each other, we both stuck to our guns and fought endless stubborn fights. We struggled to communicate and spent a very long time trying to understand each other.

It isn't like that anymore now though.

Now we know each other, we want each other, we need each other; and we love each other.

Demi is one of the most important people in my life. The love I feel for her is unconditional, and never-ending.

My family knew I had post natal depression; they lived alongside me, knowing I had it, trying to help me.

But Demi.

Demi lived through it with me. Demi is the only one that understood.

Demi saved me from myself, on more than one occasion.

She made me the Mummy I am today, and from this moment on, I will never, ever, stop protecting her or loving her.

*****

I've put the whirlpool on in the bathroom and Demi is hysterical in the bath. At first the bubbles scare her and she jumps up on to my lap, splashing as she moves and Dino and I are laughing because it's so funny to watch and soon she is giggling too, because now she finds it funny and she's jumping up and down in the water, loving it all so much and I think my cheeks are hurting from smiling so much but I don't even care because now

I feel so happy inside like nothing could spoil this perfect moment and I look back over at Dino bouncing Scotty on his lap; he too is kicking his legs about, laughing at his big sister, excited to come in and join us and my heart is just bursting with love.

We wrap them up in soft towels, drying their beautiful skin and we cradle them, holding them in to us, kissing their foreheads; stroking their gorgeous golden locks and we look at each other with such love and pride in our eyes and in our hearts and I know I am ok now. I know I am happy and my family is safe. I don't feel scared anymore. I don't feel afraid or insecure. I feel nothing but joy and happiness and I look down at my girl. My beautiful little girl; and my heart seems to hurt; ache with this new emotion; this love that fills it almost to bursting point.

\*\*\*\*\*

It's a gorgeous day today. It always seems to be hot and sunny now.

I'm at the park with the kids and with Mum. Jo and Skip are here; Dino and the babies. The sun is shining, reflecting its yellow glow on the river we now sit beside.

Demi and Ady are running and laughing; Skip and Dino kick the ball along the soft grass to my son and he squeals with delight at the fun.

We sit on the bench, the three of us. Jo, Mum and I, and my heart feels full with pride and with love. Jo is holding Franky in her arms; the image of the brother in law I now feel so close to. And Mum is between us; holding our hands in hers; smiling while she watches the kids.

I know now, that the only person missing is my Father. The Daddy I have always loved; cherished more than I could ever tell him. And I miss him; because he should be here; sharing these moments with us; before it's too late.

But I put these thoughts aside, and concentrate on who is here; the rest of the family I love and adore.

Dino pushes Scotty on the swing; I can see his huge cheeky grin from across the park and I feel my eyes prickling with tears; new tears; happy tears.

I'm forcing them away though; because I don't need to cry today.

Today my eyes have opened to a new world; a place I deserve to be, that I had hidden from, for so long.

So I squeeze my Mothers hand tighter and glance at my darling sister; marvelling at how she holds her youngest son; such a beautiful sight to my eyes. No envy now; just pride.

And I watch Mum rise; run after her only granddaughter; both of them smiling and giggling.

Soon we are moving; all walking alongside each other; towards the river bank and the wooden tables we can sit at.

Dino and Skip walk our children to the café; treat them to ice creams that will just end up all over their faces, and we sit again, with the babies, watching the water and the boats and the sun shining from the sky above, and I smile; like now I can't stop.

Because now I know it's over. All the bad feelings have gone, and I'm left only with happiness and with joy and I hug my arms around myself; like I want to contain this feeling and never let it go.

*****

I'm ok now; I'm finally ok. I don't have the evil thoughts

now, or the terror of the evil man coming for me. I know I'm safe now; safe at my Daddy's house, with my darling Dino and my beautiful babies; close to the Mother I thought I had lost.

And I love them now; all of them, like I never thought I would.

I see how my life has changed; how I've grown and strengthened as a person. My plans in life have changed too. There's so much more I want to do; so much inside I have to give.

That's why I sponsor my boy in Thailand; send him money every month for his education and write to him to help him grieve for the Mummy he has lost.

I give everything I can to charities that need it more than I ever could. Money has never meant much to me, and I doubt it ever will. What I have; I will now always give.

I have plans to travel when my babies are older. I want to see the world; help in orphanages in Africa and visit children in poverty in Thailand.

I'm going to work in support groups for mothers who have been or who are suffering from post-natal depression and will let them lean on me as much as they need to.

Because although Post-Natal Depression changed my life forever; I plan to bring something positive back from it.

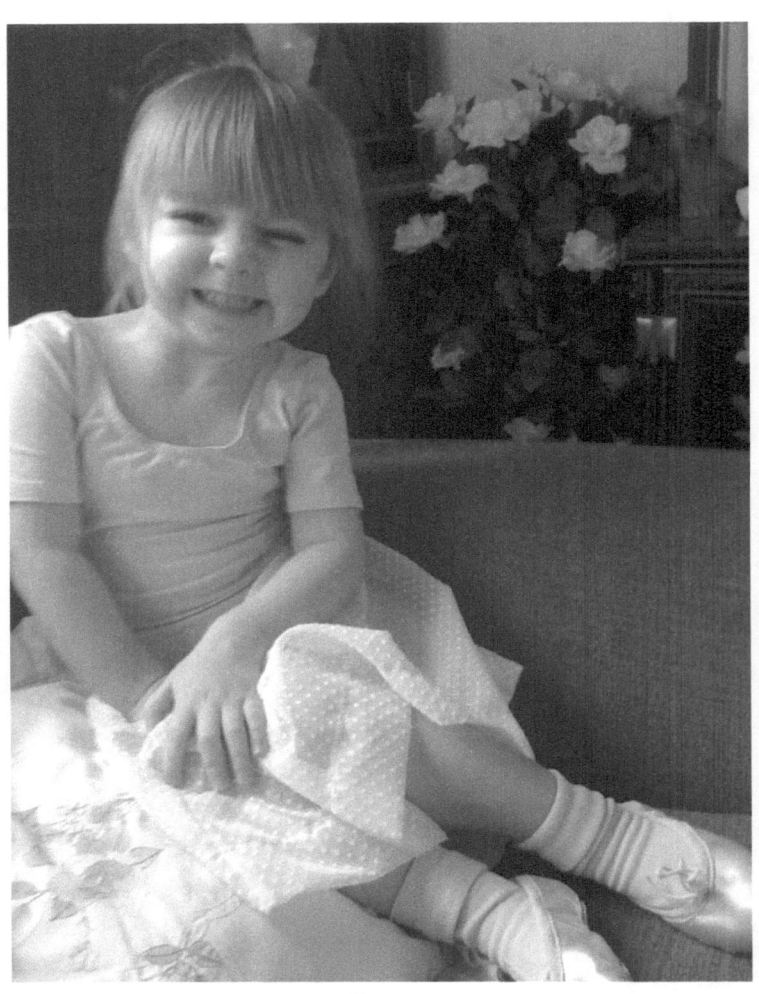

Demi

# Help

When I first felt the symptoms of post-natal depression;
I thought I was alone and going crazy.
That wasn't entirely true though!

Apparently 10 in every 100 women can develop this
illness after the birth of their babies.
It is so important to get help.
Initially it seems impossible; unthinkable to discuss those
private emotions and feelings with anyone else; let alone
a stranger.
But sometimes it's necessary.
It might help to keep a diary of how you're feeling. If you
look back over time you can see how your feelings are
changing; if the medication you might need to be on is
helping or if it isn't strong enough.

Originally I didn't want to go on tablets. I was worried
that they can often make things worse, as some anti-
depressants can make you feel suicidal, and so at first I
had counselling.
I saw a specific counsellor for my miscarriages and then
over time saw psychologists.
Personally I was not comfortable discussing things with
them.
It helps many people though and if it is what you need

then speak to your doctor.

GP's deal with things like post-natal depression on a regular basis and can probably understand your feelings far more than anybody else.

None of my family were prepared for what happened; we weren't expecting it and had no idea how to deal with it. It is really important to deal with the feelings though; however impossible it seems.

If you think/know you have post-natal depression but don't feel strong enough to talk about it with a partner/ relative, let them read this book, or one like it.
I printed web pages off for Dino and my parents, and let them read for themselves how I was likely to be feeling.
If I tried to speak about what was going on in my head; I'd freeze up and literally start to wretch.
It was as if thousands of words wanted to jump out of my mouth all at the same time; but they couldn't. Like there was a huge solid lump in my throat; blocking my voice; choking me if I tried.
The most important thing to remember is that it doesn't last forever.
It doesn't go away for many women in a matter of weeks; it is long lasting and it's very difficult to cope with, but it doesn't kill you; it doesn't really poison your body.
There is not an evil being inside you like I believed there was.
Unfortunately, it is tricks the mind chooses to play on you.
You need to be smart and try and contain how you're

feeling to a degree.

You don't need to hurt yourself; punishing your body really doesn't help in the long run. My scars are just a constant reminder; I didn't gain anything from them.
I believe that suffering from post-natal depression does completely and utterly change your life and the lives of the people you're closest to.

I'll never be the person I used to be, but Dino and I deal with the Rachel I am now. He said he has never stopped loving me; the love just grew and deepened.

If I had to advise anyone with post-natal depression; I would ask them, no, wait; beg them, not to hide.

Tell someone; anyone, how you are feeling, and then the pain will ease.

Some websites can be really helpful and often have chat forums where you can talk to other mums/parents about how you are feeling.

Some of the sites I used were:

www.netmums.com
www.bounty.com
www.patient.co.uk
www.healthcarea2z.org

I recently created a website of my own:
www.pndrachelday.com